ON
PACE

DISCOVER HOW TO RUN
EVERY RACE
AT YOUR REAL LIMIT

Matt Fitzgerald

—— 80/20 ——
p u b l i s h i n g

——— 80/20 ———
p u b l i s h i n g

80/20 Publishing, LLC
1916 N 1150 E
Lehi, UT 84043
www.8020books.com

Library of Congress Control Number: 2021952490
ISBN 979-8-9853980-0-7 (paperback)
ISBN 979-8-9853980-1-4 (e-book)
Cover and interior design by Hopewell Design
Cover photo: AP Photo/Elise Amendola

Contents

For Bob, Cat, Katie,
Pathik, Roger, and Suzanna

———————

66

It is a misconception to think that during evolution
humans sacrificed physical skill in exchange for intelligence:
wielding one's body is a mental activity."

—TED CHIANG, "UNDERSTAND"

1

Why Pacing Matters

The men's elite competition at the 2019 Berlin Marathon was not set up as a formal world record attempt. In prior years it had been, and with good success. Eight of the previous ten men's marathon world records had been recorded in Berlin, including the existing record of 2:01:39 set by Eliud Kipchoge the year before. The marquee entrant in 2019 was Kenenisa Bekele, widely considered the greatest distance runner God ever created but who, at thirty-seven, was getting a bit long in the tooth and was three years past his last major victory. Hired pacers had been asked to take the race out at 2:55 per kilometer (about 4:41 per mile), which would yield a fast but not historically fast marathon time, close to Bekele's personal best (PB) of 2:03:03 if sustained for the full 42.2 kilometers. Prevailing opinion in online fan forums was that Bekele himself would not only fail to sustain it but fail to finish, as he'd done in two of his last four marathons.

On the eve of the event, the soft-spoken Ethiopian told the assembled media, "Overall I have prepared well, although my training period of three months is perhaps rather short for a marathon. This was because of an earlier injury. But I am ready for Sunday and want to show what I can do." Having followed Bekele's career closely from the time he burst onto the international running scene with an astonishing 33-second win at the 2001 IAAF Junior World Cross Country Championships, I read more into these last few words than the more casual fan might. To me, they signaled that Bekele intended to run very fast indeed, and that he wished to show one man in particular "what he could do."

Eliud Kipchoge and Kenenisa Bekele had been rivals since 2003, when the latter nipped the former by 0.35 second in a 5000-meter race in Oslo. The pair had met again nineteen times thereafter, Bekele coming out ahead in thirteen of these races but losing all four of the marathons they'd started together. Now in the twilight of his illustrious career, Bekele might have had his last chance to cross a finish line in front of his Kenyan nemesis, but taking down his world record would certainly qualify as the next best thing.

My interpretation of Bekele's pre-race comments was validated the next morning when a small lead pack headed by a pair of striped-vested pacers passed through 5 km in 14:24, well ahead of the stated pace and precisely matching Kipchoge's split from the previous year. In the center of the scrum, a relaxed Bekele looked almost as if he were napping on his feet, waiting for the *real* start of the race. When you've watched a runner compete as many times as I've watched Bekele, you can tell by the subtlest cues if he's got his best stuff on a given day, and I could tell by Bekele's half-lidded eyes that he had good legs on this particular day, and knew it.

A shrunken lead group passed through 10 km 1 second ahead of Kipchoge's record pace and remained a single tick to the good at the halfway point. I knew this could be no accident. Bekele was going for it! The problem, though, was that Kipchoge had sped up significantly in the second half of his record-breaking performance, and Bekele would have to do the same to snatch the coveted title from his rival. Yet Bekele continued to snooze even after the pacers peeled off, leaving him with only a pair of less heralded compatriots to share the work, and by the time they reached 25 km, the Ethiopian trio had fallen 6 seconds behind the invisible specter of Kipchoge.

Approaching 30 km, and another 4 seconds off Kipchoge's standard, twenty-five-year-old Birhanu Legese launched an attack of his own. Sisay Lemma covered it quickly, but Bekele was gapped. Grimacing, he locked his now wide-open eyes on Legese's back like the threat it was, skipping his next drink bottle to save the fraction of a second that grabbing it would have cost him, but it was no use. The aggressor continued to pull away, shaking off Lemma within a few blocks on his way to passing 35 km with a 13-second advantage on the greatest of all time.

The thing is, Bekele hadn't actually slowed down. In fact, he hit 35 km having recorded his own fastest 5K split of the day, and the grimace was gone.

A nervous glance back from Legese affirmed what, by then, Bekele already understood—the younger man was faltering. Bekele came after him like an assassin. Alone in my home office in California, I began to holler at my computer screen.

Just past 37 km, Bekele overtook Legese with brutal authority, as though the would-be usurper were already forgotten, which in fact he was. Back on world record pace, Bekele was now chasing someone else, present but unseen.

The next 12 minutes were as thrilling as any athletic spectacle I've witnessed. A famously beautiful runner, Bekele ran more beautifully than I could ever hope to describe in those last few solitary minutes on Berlin's Teutonically perfect streets, his trademark sprinter's back kick in full effect, head rocking ever so slightly in small concession to fatigue, checking his watch frequently, as though he heard the television commentators raving about how close it was going to be.

More than beautiful, Bekele's self-sacrificial charge to the finish line was *heroic*, the stuff of legend, an aging champion's all-costs bid to etch one last triumph into his legacy. Bekele shot through Brandenburg Gate at 2:00:39 on the race clock, leaving precisely 1 minute to close the deal. The crowd waiting on the other side went berserk. Wincing with effort, Bekele tried to accelerate but couldn't, for he was already sprinting and had been for some time. The video feed now switched to a camera stationed behind the finish line. I saw Bekele grinding. I saw the clock, ticking up, counting down. It was impossible to judge the distance. Could he do it? 2:01:31, 32, 33 . . .

Two seconds. He missed by 2 seconds! That's 0.02 percent. Yet Bekele was far from disappointed by the oh-so-near miss. "I knew I was very close to the record but I couldn't quite make it," he told reporters at a post-race press conference. "Before the race, I did not expect a world record, so I am very happy to take 80 seconds off my personal best."

As a fan of elite running, I love this performance for its poetry and drama. But as a coach, I see it as the epitome of skillful pacing.

THE QUINTESSENTIAL RUNNING SKILL

Pacing is *the art of finding your limit*. Harder than it looks, this quintessential running skill is supported by three key aptitudes: body awareness, judgment, and toughness.

Body awareness (or what scientists call somatic awareness) relates to a runner's feel for her performance limits. Although pacing can be assisted by objective data (as evidenced by Bekele's frequent watch glances), it is done mainly by feel. All competitive runners share a common goal of reaching the finish line in the least time possible. Throughout each race, a single question looms: *Can I sustain this effort level for the remaining distance?* The answer comes not in the form of numbers or words but as perceptions, a continuous evaluation of present levels of effort and fatigue in relation to past experience. That same looming question could also be formulated this way: *Am I feeling how I should be feeling at this point of the race?*

Some runners are better than others at reading these perceptions, and Bekele showed exquisite sensitivity to his limits in Berlin, most obviously when he held steady instead of answering Legese's attack, but not only then. When Bekele said after the race that he did not expect a world record, I took him at his word. Why, then, did he start the marathon smack on record pace? Because every pacing master knows better than to allow expectations to rule his performance. Goals and expectations provide a good starting point for successful race execution, but that's all they do. When the gun goes off and you start moving, you need to be willing and able to adjust your effort appropriately based on external conditions and also on disparities between how you expected to feel and how you actually feel.

For the runner, such adjustments can go in either of two directions. While it's more common to sense the need to dial back one's effort from the expected or desired pace in response to adverse conditions or shaky legs, there are occasional, special races in which the perceptive runner discovers that he is capable of something remarkable, as Bekele did in Berlin. But a single early adjustment is not enough. Optimal pacing is a matter of incessant fine-tuning, as Bekele demonstrated in taking full advantage of the opportunity he discerned when he came out the other side of his rough patch.

Which brings us to judgment. Bekele's decision to let Legese and Lemma get away from him between 30 and 37 km was just that: a decision, and one that not every runner would have made. In his post-race remarks, Bekele revealed that his left hamstring had tightened up when he'd tried to answer Legese's surge, hence the grimace. Although frustrated by the ill-timed anatomical malfunction, Bekele knew better than to resist it, so he shifted his focus from staying with the leader to limiting his losses and remaining in a position to take advantage of Legese's faltering, should it happen. And it did happen, because Legese had made a mistake—specifically, a pacing mistake—in surging too hard too early in the race. In fact, he wound up finishing more than a minute behind his elder.

To fully capitalize on the opportunity his body awareness and judgment had created, Bekele needed to exercise the third key aptitude for pacing mastery: toughness. Most runners are tough, but Bekele demonstrated a rare kind of toughness in going after Kipchoge's world record in the "I-don't-care-how-much-it-hurts" manner that he did. There is no way to objectively measure how hard one is trying in a race. A runner might feel she tried as hard as she could in a race only to plunge even deeper into the pain cave in the next one, when perhaps there's more at stake. In running, the limit is always mental, the pain tank always filling before the gas tank empties, and the tougher a runner is, the closer she can get to her unreachable physical limit before she hits her invisible, but no less real, mental limit.

In addition to showing us what good pacing looks like, Bekele's stunning return to glory in Berlin teaches us how much good pacing matters. At the professional level today, even the marathon is a game of seconds. As painful as it must have been for Bekele to fall 2 measly seconds short of setting a world record, I doubt he was able, in looking back on the race, to come up with a single alternative tactical decision that would have gained him the mite of time he needed to make history. Which is my point—that it is possible to become so good at pacing that you can't find one solid reason to think you could have done even 0.02 percent better.

I used to coach a runner named Chris whose personal-best marathon time prior to hiring me was 3:13. When it came time for his next marathon, Chris was in 3:05 shape, but he ended up running 3:08 after having completed the first 20 miles at 3:02 pace and then blowing up. As a general matter, I am happy with an athlete's race performance whenever the athlete himself is happy, but in this case, I must admit I was a little unhappy when, after having wasted roughly 3.2 percent of his fitness, Chris texted me to say he felt good about losing "only a few minutes" in the last few miles.

"A few minutes!" I wanted to reply (but didn't). "Is that your idea of good pacing?"

HOW I CAME TO KNOW THE POWER OF PACING

My earliest memory of running "long distance" dates back to 1978, when I was seven years old and living with my family in the deep woods of Hillsboro, New Hampshire. My dad, who at that time ran for fitness (he would later become a marathoner), owned a cool little gadget that he would hook to the waistband of his shorts and use to measure distance when he "jogged" (his word). This pedometer, as it was called, looked like a cross between a compass and a pocket watch and made a satisfying clicking sound with each stride. I had no particular interest in jogging at that age, but I was very interested in Dad's pedometer, so I took it for a test drive one day, clicking off a full mile (assuming the thing was accurate).

By the age of twelve, under my father's continued influence, I was running regularly, using a cheap children's sports watch to measure time and using various landmarks—mapped out with the aid of the family's Renault odometer—for distance. Numbers weren't the be-all and end-all of the running experience for me, but I liked how they gave purpose to it. A soccer player as well, I saw times and distances as being roughly equivalent to the tally of goals and assists I kept as a striker for the Bobcats of Oyster River Middle School.

In high school, having been forced to quit soccer after I suffered a catastrophic knee injury during a game, I ran cross country and track. Our team's bread-and-butter track workout during the outdoor season was 12 × 400 meters at roughly 1-mile race pace. My teammates and I made a game of it, each runner taking his turn leading a lap, at the completion of which the others tried to guess the time. We got so good at the game that the winning guess was seldom more than a few tenths off in either direction.

More than a decade later, at twenty-eight, I ran my first half marathon in runway-flat Phoenix. In addition to the usual awards for overall and age-group placement, a prize was given by the race organizer to the runner who came closest to correctly predicting his or her finish time. I reckoned I was fit enough to average 6:00 per mile, which would yield a finish time of 1:18:39. To take a bit of pressure off myself, I rounded up to 1:19:00, which was unfortunate because my actual time of 1:18:46 would have earned me a gift certificate from a local running specialty shop.

A short time later I started coaching other runners. Like a lot of new coaches, I took my own depth of experience for granted initially. Forgetting I hadn't always known how to pace my running effectively, I was surprised by the kinds of mistakes my clients made. The biggest one I saw was getting stuck in what I call the moderate-intensity rut—doing way too much training in the no-man's-land between easy and hard. I've since become known for advocating an "80/20" training method, where 80 percent of training is consciously performed at low intensity and the rest at moderate to high intensity.

I also saw plenty of clients making the same mistake that Chris made in his marathon: bad pacing. It's really two mistakes in one, both of which are reflected in his example. The first is poor execution, as evidenced by Chris's hot start and late-race unraveling. The second is failure to value pacing properly, as revealed by the way Chris shrugged off the loss of "a few minutes" in our post-marathon debriefing. Imagine a boxer shrugging off having taken a few extra punches to the head that might have been avoided with more vigilant defenses, or a golfer shrugging off a few quadruple bogeys that might have been avoided with more careful club selection!

COMPETE AT YOUR FULL POTENTIAL

Pacing is everything in competitive distance running. I mean it: everything. It is the sport's defining characteristic—the singular quiddity that makes distance running different from all other sports and exercise activities, including other forms of running. Take sprinting. The word "sprint" is used rather loosely in colloquial speech, but the true definition of a sprint is a race that is performed at maximal effort from start to finish, which is to say without pacing. By this standard, there is no such thing as a sprint that lasts longer than 45 seconds, give or take, because it is not physically possible to sustain a maximal effort longer than approximately 45 seconds. It is pacing that distinguishes a distance event from a sprint (a race that lasts longer than a maximal effort can be sustained from a race that doesn't). At the other extreme is jogging, or running for exercise, as my dad used to do in his pedometer days. Jogging is also a form of running, but we don't lump it together with the sport of distance running any more than we do sprinting. The difference again is pacing. In this case, whereas the noncompetitive jogger is just trying to fill a certain amount of time with healthy exertion, the competitive distance runner is trying to cover a fixed distance in the least time possible, an objective that demands skillful pacing.

Naturally, some competitive runners are more serious than others, but every runner should take pacing seriously and seek to master the skill. It's a very different sort of commitment than spending thousands of dollars on gear or working out twice a day every day. You don't have to carve out extra time or accept a higher risk of injury to get serious about becoming a pacing master. Like a boxer staying vigilant in his defenses or a golfer taking pains to always select the right club for the next shot, a runner should make every reasonable effort to ensure bad pacing doesn't needlessly limit their improvement. Do you really want to run slower race times than you could just because you can't be bothered to master your sport's most fundamental skill? I didn't think so!

For me, though, pacing's importance goes even deeper. I see it as a democratizing element of our sport. There's nothing you can do about your talent. Whatever genes you were born with, those are the genes you have to work with. But pacing skill is a completely different matter that depends on body awareness, judgment, and toughness—qualities that aren't affected one way or the other by innate ability. Sure, Kenenisa Bekele happens to have all of these things, including raw talent, in abundance, but there are plenty of runners with far less talent who possess just as much of the other three qualities. Indeed, there's no reason the slowest runner in a given race can't be the best pacer. Nor is there any reason you can't find the absolute limit of your potential by mastering the skill of pacing.

Every runner stops getting faster at some point. But pacing is something that any runner can get better at indefinitely, which is kind of cool. No matter how well you executed your last race, there's always a chance you can do even better the next time. So if you're the kind of runner who likes to improve, know that pacing is the one part of running you can improve in for as long as you choose to run.

I'll give you an example from my own running. In March of 2020 I returned home to California from a trip to Atlanta with an infection that I later discovered was COVID-19. I was sick for an entire month and lost a ton of fitness.

When I was finally well enough to run again, I decided to participate in a virtual marathon that was then just six and a half weeks away. I knew I couldn't attain peak fitness in such a limited amount of time, but I was curious to see how much progress I could achieve by making full use of my decades of experience.

In a normal training cycle, by the time race day comes around I have a good feel for how fit I am and what sort of performance I am capable of, so I know how to pace myself. But this was not a normal training cycle. As experienced as I was, the situation I found myself in as I approached the Rambling Runner Virtual Marathon was novel in many respects. I wasn't sure how fit I was, and I could only guess how fast I was ready to run. But there's a difference between uncertainty and utter cluelessness, and my forty-five-day buildup gave me enough clues to enable me to set a goal that, while not as sure a bet as my typical race goal, wasn't completely arbitrary either. The plan I came up with was to run the first 10K at 6:49 per mile (setting myself up for a sub-3-hour finish, barring disaster), then reassess and go from there.

I started out a little hot, completing the first mile in 6:44. Had I truly *known* that 6:49 per mile was the fastest pace I could sustain for the full marathon distance, I would at that point have made the necessary correction. But my body was telling me something else, and having completed more than fifty marathons, I knew I could trust it. Long story short, I went on to complete the marathon in 2:54:42, averaging 6:40 per mile for the full distance. My half-marathon splits were 1:27:51 and 1:26:41. My last two full miles were my fastest, but not by much—6:29 and 6:31—indicating nearly flawless pacing. I neither ran out of gas before I finished, nor finished with gas left in the tank, but instead ran out of gas *as I finished*.

It wasn't my fastest marathon, but it was perhaps my most satisfying. In the final analysis, the time on the clock means nothing. What matters is how you got there. How closely does that time match the best you could have done with perfect execution, including flawless mastery of the pacing process? When I ran my lifetime-best marathon in Chicago three years earlier, I finished knowing I could have gone a little faster. But when I completed the Rambling Runner Virtual Marathon alone in my quiet suburban neighborhood, I did so knowing I had realized very nearly 100 percent of my potential on the day, and it felt fantastic. And I want you to experience that same feeling.

As I've stated, most runners are not very good at pacing. Why not? I'll provide a fuller answer to this question in Chapter 3, but here are the three main reasons:

1. Pacing is hard! Nobody is great at it initially.
2. Experience is the best teacher of pacing skill, and most runners lack the depth of experience that enables pacing masters to perform masterfully.
3. Runners are exceedingly dependent on their devices and this dependency hinders the development of body awareness, impedes the application of good judgment, and prevents many runners from fully accessing their toughness.

The last of these reasons is the one that really bugs me, in part because it is literally man-made, hence unnecessary, in part because it's getting worse all the time, and in part because I feel somewhat responsible. I've mentioned that I advocate an 80/20 training method as a corrective for the common problem of doing too much training at moderate intensity—which is in essence a pacing error. The method laid out in the books *80/20 Running* and *80/20 Triathlon* and on 8020endurance.com has helped tens of thousands of athletes all over the world break free of the moderate-intensity rut. Devices such as heart rate monitors and power meters are helpful in this process because they allow athletes to objectively monitor their exercise intensity, making it easier for those who aren't as adept at reading their effort by feel to balance their training intensities appropriately. The problem is that these same athletes risk becoming even more device dependent and less capable of regulating their effort by feel. This wouldn't be a big deal, I suppose, if the devices were as good at making pacing decisions as a human pacing master, but they aren't, nor will they ever be.

TRAIN YOUR ABILITY TO RUN FREE

As a coach, I now place a heavy emphasis on pacing skill development. In the beginning, my method consisted of little more than chastising athletes when they blew their pacing in a workout and patting them on the back when they did better. An admonishment to "try harder next time" was the nearest thing I had to a pacing skill development program. After all, I had come of age at a time when pacing wasn't really talked about much because lack of pacing skill wasn't a widespread problem. When the topic did come up with coaches, their stock advice was to relax and let experience take care of it. But with today's device dependency, experience isn't quite the teacher it once was. Recognizing this, I began to put a lot of thought into devising ways to counteract the negative effects of device usage on pacing skill development.

My modus operandi in all of my efforts to elevate my coaching game is to borrow from the best. Heck, even the 80/20 method that I've gotten so much mileage out of can be attributed to its discoverer, exercise physiologist Stephen Seiler (who very graciously wrote the foreword to *80/20 Triathlon*). Hence, my quest to become a better pacing teacher has largely taken the form of an ongoing effort to collect information about the things true pacing masters do that other runners don't, and to formulate these observations into techniques and practices that my athletes can implement in workouts and races. I've also delved deeply into the science of pacing, mining it for other tools with potential usefulness in the development of pacing skill. Over time, this grab bag of methods has evolved into a coherent approach to mastering pacing.

If I were a more profit-seeking and less honest person, I would tell you that this approach works perfectly in every case—that it transforms even the most inept pacer into a Bekele-level master in a matter of weeks. The truth is, it doesn't. Like every other skill, pacing ability is not distributed equally across the population. Individual athletes improve by different amounts with the same approach. But I can say that *everyone* I work with on pacing does improve, and by a greater amount, I believe, than they would by continuing to muddle along heuristically. And some do in fact achieve full mastery.

What's more, runners of all types enjoy the process. Analytical types who love data enjoy the pursuit of pacing mastery because through it they learn how to use device data more judiciously, and also how to use their own perceptions as an additional source of reliable data. Intuitive types who are daunted by technology enjoy the process because it puts them in control of their devices, which become facilitators of, rather than rivals to, their preferred run-by-feel approach. Even those whose progress comes slowly find the intentional pacing practice I guide them through makes their running more engaging and rewarding. Indeed, from my perspective as a coach, the most satisfying part of the process isn't seeing athletes get better at pacing, but watching them start to trust themselves more. Coaching legend Vern Gambetta once tweeted, "The goal in coaching is to develop self-sufficient, adaptable athletes prepared to thrive in the competitive cauldron. Give your athletes the mental and physical skills. Get them to the point where they trust in their preparation and let them go." I couldn't agree more, and in today's environment I've come to see the teaching of pacing skill as critical to achieving this larger goal.

The key concepts at play here are *self-trust* and *self-sufficiency*. There is no better feeling in the sport of running than that of knowing what you can do and then going out and doing it. That is the feeling I experienced in my post-coronavirus solo marathon, and that is what I want for you. It is fundamentally a feeling of freedom or independence, a calm confidence born of not having to rely on a watch or a coach or luck or anything else outside of yourself to find your real limit. This is what pacing skill makes possible: the power to run free.

A writer at heart, I couldn't possibly remain content with sharing what I've learned about pacing skill development with only the handful of athletes I coach one-on-one. Inevitably, I got the itch to compose a book on the subject, and here it is. My hope and expectation is that *On Pace* will do the same thing for you that my hands-on pacing guidance has done for the individual athletes I coach. I'll start out by describing the science of pacing, so you'll have a better understanding of what it means to master the skill. I will then explain more fully the specific obstacles you'll need to overcome to get where you want to go, and the most effective ways to overcome them. Next, we'll explore what it looks like to reach the other side of these obstacles—to become a pacing master. The second half of the book gets down to brass tacks, offering specific strategies, exercises, and plans you can use to programmatically improve your pacing in races, workouts, and the training process as a whole.

What this book will not do is solve the pacing problem for you. There is no silver bullet where pacing is concerned. Remember, the desire to have someone or something else do the hard work of pacing for you is what got you into this mess! You simply cannot become a pacing master without taking responsibility for it. Good coaching can help, and technology has a valid role to play as well, but in the end it's on you to execute.

There are two ways to look at this responsibility. From one perspective, it's an intimidating burden, but from another it's an opportunity. The very fact that skillful pacing is hard, and that most runners suck at it and wish someone or something else would handle it for them, creates an opening for you to become better at it than most of your fellow runners. While others remain resigned to mediocre or poor pacing or vainly hope that they'll get better at it without making any systematic effort to do so, you can leave them behind (literally) by embracing the process I'm about to teach you. I can't make any promises about how far you will get toward total freedom as a runner, but I can promise that you won't regret the journey.

2

The Science of Pacing

As much as I would like to say I wrote the book on pacing, that honor belongs to Andrew Edwards and Remco Polman, who coauthored *Pacing in Sport and Exercise* in 2011. I did, however, write the foreword to this groundbreaking volume, which I was privileged to read ahead of its public release. More than a decade later, I'm still able to recite from memory the authors' definition of pacing: "the goal-directed distribution and management of effort across the duration of an exercise bout." There's a lot packed into this short statement, including concepts of self-regulation and effort perception that are well worth exploring in depth. But first let's talk about the "goal-directed" part.

Since the beginning, scientific efforts to understand pacing have focused on the concept of the limit, and rightly so. All types of human performance, including running, are defined by their limiters. To understand what stops people from going faster, higher, or farther than they do is to understand how they go as fast, as high, and as far as they do. The thing that makes running, and especially distance running, different from other types of human performance is that the nature of the limiter is not self-evident. In a sprint, the limiter is seemingly obvious: speed. One can dig a little deeper and ask whether sprint performance is limited by how quickly an athlete can turn over her legs or by how much directional force she can apply to the ground with her foot, but such questions are answered relatively easily (turns out, it's the latter). In longer events, the limit is a lot fuzzier. At almost any point in a 1-mile track race or a 100-mile trail ultramarathon, a runner could, if he chose to, run faster than he is. So it's not a speed issue. But if not that, then what? Answering this question is key to unlocking the mystery of pacing. All runners seek their performance limit in races. Pacing is the tool we use to find our limit. But what the heck is the limiter?

IN SEARCH OF THE LIMIT

Science is essentially a formalized effort to overcome bias. It's an effort that never fully succeeds, however, because science is practiced by the same biased humans who seek to overcome their natural biases in practicing it. The quest to understand pacing has been tainted by two biases in particular. The first is an abiding tendency to privilege the physical (i.e., the body) over the nonphysical (the mind). The second is a propensity to overlook the non-measurable or not-yet-measurable in favor of the measurable. If not for these twin biases, scientists might have solved the mystery of pacing more than a century earlier than they did.

The first modern theory of human endurance was entirely biological in nature, overlooking the mind altogether. Its creator was Archibald Vivian Hill, who published under the name A. V. Hill and is widely regarded as the father of exercise science. Born in 1886 in Bristol, England, and educated at Cambridge University (where he also ran track), Hill began to study the physiology of muscle contractions in 1909. His interest in the phenomenon was sparked by the then-recent discovery that muscles have the ability to contract without a supply of oxygen. Prior to this discovery, oxygen was believed to be an absolute requirement for muscle contraction. Hill's work took the newfound existence of anaerobic (meaning "without oxygen") muscle metabolism as its starting point and yielded many additional discoveries.

In the early 1920s, Hill came up with the concept of oxygen debt, for which he was awarded a Nobel Prize. His key insight was that, although the muscles are able to perform a limited amount of work in the absence of oxygen by turning glycogen (the storage form of glucose in the muscles and liver) into lactic acid, eventually this lactic acid has to be turned back into glycogen with the help of oxygen. Hill's own experience on the track (he had a PB of 4:45 in the mile) fed into this realization. He'd always wondered why his breathing rate remained elevated for a few minutes after a hard workout or race and then gradually returned to normal. The concept of oxygen debt helped explain what the body was trying to accomplish through this process.

Hill's next step was to test his insight on athletes, including himself, by tasking them to run around an 85-meter track while breathing into a mask that collected exhaled gases in a bag worn like a backpack. The specific protocol Hill devised required subjects to go faster and faster until they reached exhaustion, a type of endurance test that became known as an open loop because there was no predetermined endpoint. Through such experiments, Hill learned that each person has a maximal rate of oxygen consumption that is highly correlated with his maximal sustained running speed. Today we refer to this limit as aerobic capacity, or VO_2max. All runners consume more oxygen as they run faster, and the fastest runners are able to consume the most oxygen, but even they reach a limit eventually, and exhaustion soon follows.

Hill pegged the heart muscle as the source of this limit. When intense exercise is sustained, he believed, the heart can't supply enough oxygen to the working muscles to meet their energy needs, causing the muscles to make up the balance by turning glycogen into lactic acid without oxygen. But only so much oxygen debt and lactic acid can accumulate before the muscles fail, at which point the athlete must slow down or stop so that oxygen can be made available in sufficient quantities to turn the accumulated lactic acid back into glycogen.

Hill now stood just one small step away from formulating a theory of pacing. He had identified the limiter of endurance exercise—or so he thought. All that was left for him to do was to figure out how athletes manage to reach but not exceed their limit in competition. Oddly, Hill never took this final step. The reason, I suspect, has to do with the open-loop nature of Hill's experiments, where subjects ran at incrementally increasing speeds to the point of failure. This format made sense in that it was the failure point that Hill was most interested in. He wanted to know what caused an athlete to stop when he did. The problem, however, was that there was no self-pacing element in this protocol. The pace was set by the experimenter, not the runner, who was required to keep accelerating on command until he couldn't. This is completely different from an actual race, which is a closed-loop endurance test where each athlete regulates his own pace. Steeped as Hill was in his experimental design, it seems to have never crossed his mind to explain how pacing operated in relation to the hard limit of muscle failure.

Fortunately, the next generation of exercise scientists stepped up to develop a theory of pacing that was consistent with Hill's biological explanation of human endurance. Less fortunately, it wasn't a very good theory. What these mid-century bioreductionists proposed was that athletes somehow automatically race at the highest speed they can sustain without causing their muscles to fail before they reach the finish line. A key contributor to this literally mindless theory of pacing was David Costill, who did his most important work at Ball State University in Muncie, Indiana. In 1978, Costill led an experiment in which lactic acid levels were measured in eighteen runners as they completed time trials and races of various distances ranging from 3.2 kilometers to a marathon. As expected, lactic acid levels were found to be higher in shorter events run at faster speeds and lower in longer events run at lower speeds. At all distances, however, performance was highly correlated with the subjects' maximal lactate steady state (MLSS) running speed, or the highest speed each runner was able to sustain in a separate test without going into oxygen debt. On the basis of this finding, Costill's team concluded that "runners may set a race pace which closely approximates the running velocity at which lactate begins to accumulate."

Absent from this study was any effort to explain how runners identify the velocity at which lactate begins to accumulate. One thing is certain: Runners don't wear lactate meters that enable them to stay just below the allowable limit in the same way that motorists use their speedometer to stay below the legal speed limit. This left only two possibilities, assuming Costill's speculation was correct. One was that the brain possessed some sort of hidden internal lactate meter that monitored blood lactate and enforced a limit in the way a thermostat enforces a temperature limit. The other was blind trial and error—an unconstrained process whereby runners find out the hard way how fast they can go without exceeding the lactate limit at each race distance. Neither of these possibilities had any empirical backing. People don't *feel* their blood lactate level the way they feel other things, like body temperature. And as for the second possibility, while it is true that most runners are bad at pacing initially and get better over time, they aren't nearly as bad as we would expect them to be if their pacing decisions were entirely a matter of trial and error.

Another problem with Costill's conclusion that lactic acid accumulation limits performance at a range of exercise intensities is the fact that, as Costill himself observed, lactic acid levels vary widely in races of different distances. If lactic acid really caused muscle failure, it would do so at one specific level. In response to this criticism, believers in a strictly biological model of endurance broadened it to encompass other mechanisms of fatigue. The revised explanation of pacing that came out of this effort proposed that fatigue was caused by different mechanisms in different situations. In a short test lasting only a few minutes, for example, fatigue might be caused by muscle cell depolarization (the same mechanism that causes batteries to fail), whereas in a longer test it might be caused by a core body temperature increase or muscle damage or glycogen depletion.

What did not change in this modified model, however, was the general idea that endurance performance was limited by physiological failure. All it did was multiply the types of failure that might occur, and in so doing it multiplied the pacing problem, offering no answer to the question of how athletes regulate their effort in such a way as to just barely avoid whichever specific type of failure would occur first in a particular event.

But there was an even bigger problem: Endurance performance is not actually limited by physiological failures of any kind. It's true that intense and prolonged exercise causes all kinds of disruptions to biological homeostasis. Lactic acid levels increase, pH levels decrease, cellular damage occurs, glycogen levels drop, core body temperature climbs, and more. But in study after study after study, researchers found that none of these disruptions ever reached a point where it could have directly forced an athlete to stop exercising involuntarily.

The final experimental nail in the coffin of the biological model of exercise tolerance came in the form of a meticulously designed study by Spanish researchers that appeared in the *Journal of Physiology* in 2015. Its aim was to exercise volunteers to the point of exhaustion in a variety of ways and measure absolutely everything to find out once and for all which specific physiological breakdown, if any, set the limit. Twenty-two subjects performed 10-second, all-out sprints on stationary bikes, recovered fully, and then pedaled at incrementally increasing power levels to failure—not once but on multiple occasions, with new wrinkles added each time. In half of the tests, the subjects breathed regular air, while in the other half they breathed oxygen-poor air, simulating high altitude.

After quitting each test, the subjects rested for either 10 seconds or 1 minute, with either a normal blood supply to the legs or a constricted blood supply, and then repeated the all-out, 10-second sprints. Among the measurements taken during and after each variation were blood lactate level, muscle pH, and ATP level (ATP being the muscle cells' fundamental energy currency).

The results showed that neither lack of energy supply to the muscles nor chemical disruptions within the muscles could explain the subjects' quitting. For example, when blood supply to the legs was constricted, the subjects were able to produce more power in a 10-second sprint after 1 minute of recovery than after 10 seconds of recovery, which one would intuitively expect. Yet lactic acid levels were higher and pH levels were lower after the longer recovery, which was a problem for the idea that either high lactic acid levels or low pH levels caused exhaustion. Having no other option, the researchers concluded, "At the end of an incremental exercise to exhaustion, a large functional reserve remains in the muscles to generate power, even at levels far above the power output at which task failure occurs."

In lay terms, this means the subjects were physically able to keep exercising at the time they stopped. There was no physiological failure. Crazy, right? But facts are facts. The great thing about science is that, although susceptible to bias, it is self-correcting. Given time, it exposes its biases, opening the door to a truer truth. To the (ironic) credit of science, exercise scientists who believed that exhaustion is caused by physiological breakdown were the ones to prove that exhaustion is not caused by physiological breakdown. Which meant that pacing could not be a physiological process. Which meant that pacing remained unexplained.

COMMON SENSE TO THE RESCUE

A. V. Hill's biological model of exercise tolerance actually fell apart long before the Spanish study just described buried it once and for all. The inability of its proponents to produce a scintilla of proof that endurance performance was limited by any specific physiological breakdown was common knowledge within the field of exercise physiology as early as the 1990s. Then, in 1996, a South African medical doctor turned exercise physiologist proposed an alternative model of exercise tolerance, which shifted the performance limiter *from the body to the brain*. Tim Noakes argued that, during exercise, the brain receives continuous feedback from various organs and systems of the body—chemical and electrical information streams that enable the brain to monitor things like core body temperature, blood glucose, and hydration; to assess the athlete's well-being from moment to moment; and to react protectively when necessary. If the feedback coming into the brain signals an impending crisis—hyperthermia, hyponatremia, or whatever—the brain, acting as a kind of governor (hence the model's name: the central governor theory), automatically reduces muscle activation, causing the athlete to slow down involuntarily. And there's your limit—not physiological failure, but *the threat* thereof.

Pacing, according to this theory, is all about anticipation. Writing in 2011, Noakes explained, "The goal of pacing is to maintain homeostasis and to prevent a catastrophic physiological failure. Multiple, independent systems in the periphery provide sensory feedback that influences central motor drive from the brain to the exercising muscles. The outcome of this information is the pacing strategy that develops during exercise." The governor, then, is a brain-based mechanism that estimates the maximum speed that can be safely sustained over an expected duration and actively enforces this limit.

The central governor theory made a huge impact, not only within exercise science but also beyond it, influencing endurance coaches and athletes all over the world. It had problems of its own, however. Some critics pointed out that if the central governor existed, then we ought to be able to find it. After all, plenty is known about which specific parts of the brain handle different functions. If you're startled by a sudden movement in the periphery of your vision, blame the amygdala. If you succeed in resisting the temptation to eat a cookie you know you don't need, credit the anterior cingulate cortex. Yet despite rapid advances in functional brain imaging and related technologies, nobody has been able to pinpoint a specific brain structure that holds runners back automatically, by just the right amount, in a race.

Another problem was that the central governor theory completely ignored a little thing called *consciousness*, assigning no role to the thoughts and perceptions we all experience in our efforts to pace our runs. To the extent that Noakes's theory made sense, it did so for zombies, not humans. In response to this second criticism, Noakes revised the theory to make space for conscious brain operations, but this only opened the door to another criticism: If pacing can't be explained without reference to conscious thoughts and perceptions, what need is there for an unconscious central governor that can't even be found?

Among Noakes's favorite "proofs" of the existence of a central governor that controls pacing was the well-known "end spurt" phenomenon, whereby athletes abruptly speed up at the end of a long race, just when (according to A. V. Hill's model of exercise tolerance) they are presumably nearest to their physical limit. Noakes was certainly right to point out that the strict biological explanation of pacing did not account for this almost universal phenomenon. But in an attention-grabbing 2008 paper published in the *European Journal of Applied Physiology*, a brash young Italian exercise scientist named Samuele Marcora challenged Noakes's own explanation of the end spurt and offered a more human, less zombielike alternative. Marcora's simpler explanation for the end spurt was that athletes use a combination of perceived exertion (aka perceived effort) and awareness of where they are within a race to make conscious pacing choices that ensure they "save something" for the end, at which point they go ahead and empty the tank. Because runners cannot precisely anticipate how things will stand near the end of a race, Marcora argued, and because finishing the race is paramount, "athletes usually choose a slightly conservative pace for most of the race. Near the end of the race, when the information provided by the conscious sensation of effort at a certain running speed is more reliable, most 'conservative' athletes realize that they can significantly increase running speed without reaching exhaustion before the finishing line, and decide to go for an end-spurt. No additional subconscious intelligent system is needed, just our conscious brain."

In 2009, one year after his editorial appeared, Marcora introduced his own theory of endurance, which he called the psychobiological model of exercise tolerance. According to this new model, the true limiter of endurance performance is neither the body's functional capacity nor a brain-based protective reflex that keeps us from exceeding our physical capacity, but conscious self-regulation, where sensations and behavior are controlled through deliberate decisions made in pursuit of goals.

In a stark break from exercise science tradition, Marcora based his model not on biochemistry but on psychology, and specifically on a construct known as motivational intensity theory. Developed by Jack Brehm in the 1980s, motivational intensity theory asserts that people enter into difficult tasks, whether physical or mental, with a certain degree of *potential motivation* that predetermines the maximal amount of effort they are willing to exert to achieve their goal. If this limit is exceeded before the goal has been achieved, they disengage. Marcora proposed that endurance racing is like any other task in that, when an athlete hits the proverbial wall in a race, it is not because the body has encountered a physical limit but rather because the athlete has decided that the effort required to keep pushing is too great. It's not that physical limits don't exist— they're just never actually encountered in the endurance context because one of two things always happens first: the goal is achieved, or the effort required to continue pursuing the goal exceeds the athlete's potential motivation and the athlete backs off, by choice.

What makes endurance exercise different from other tasks is the specific form that effort takes. In most everyday tasks, such as desk work and parenting, effort takes the form of a nebulous mix of internal resources such as concentration and willpower. In running, however, the dominant form of effort is *perceived effort*. In a 2010 paper, Samuele Marcora defined this critical concept as follows: "Perception of effort, also known as perceived exertion or sense of effort, refers to the conscious sensation of how hard, heavy, and strenuous a physical task is. This perception depends mainly on feelings of effort in the active limbs, and the sensation of heavy breathing (a type of dyspnea)." I will explain how the brain generates this perception in Chapter 6, but for now it's sufficient to note that as the intensity of running increases, and as fatigue sets in, perceived effort rises, becoming more and more uncomfortable. If running continues, the runner will eventually reach a perceived effort level that he feels is intolerable, at which point he will quit. The true limiter of endurance performance, then, is a *feeling*.

PSYCHOLOGICAL LIMITS

This is a good place to mention that it's not only scientists who tend to be dismissive of the nonphysical and nonmeasurable. We all are. We are therefore prone to think of psychological limits as being less real than physical limits, and yet they aren't. Take pain, for example. Studies of pain tolerance have found that everyone has a limit as to how much pain they can tolerate, even when the pain they are experiencing is causing no physical harm. It's the same with perceived effort, and this is why in open-loop fitness tests, even the toughest runners step off the treadmill before they physically have to.

Psychological limits are admittedly kind of smudgy compared to physical limits. When there's more at stake, pain tolerance goes up. Similarly, when (in psychobiological terms) the potential motivation level is higher, perceived effort tolerance goes up. This has been shown in a variety of studies, including a 2012 experiment by British exercise scientists Alexis Mauger and Nick Sculthorpe in which subjects completed a pair of VO_2max tests, one of which was a standard open loop, where runners kept running faster and faster in incremental steps to failure, and the other of which was a novel closed-loop test, which was fixed at 10 minutes in length. As you will recall from earlier in the chapter, VO_2max is supposed to be a hard physiological limit, and yet the subjects of this experiment were able to achieve 8 percent higher VO_2max scores in the closed-loop test than they did in the open-loop test.

How come? Mauger and Sculthorpe speculated that the subjects were simply more motivated in the closed loop, hence they dug deeper—and I think they're right. Remember, according to Brehm's motivational intensity theory, people tend to disengage from tasks when they've either completed them successfully or when they feel that continuing is not worth the effort. In an open-loop run, there's really no such thing as successful task completion; the only thing you get for continuing to run is greater suffering. But in a 10-minute VO_2max test, you know you're done after 10 minutes no matter what, so it's easy to motivate yourself to give it all you've got.

What's important to note here is that the subjects in this study *felt* they were working as hard as they could in both tests, even though they were objectively working harder in the closed loop. It is in this sense that maximal perceived effort tolerance represents a real limit that cannot be exceeded in any circumstances, but it's a mutable limit that may align with different physiological measurements in different circumstances, depending on how they affect potential motivation.

In the years since Marcora introduced the psychobiological model of exercise tolerance, he and other scientists have gathered plenty of evidence in support of the idea that endurance races are indeed paced by perceived effort. One example is a study led by Bruno Ferreira Viana of the University of Rio de Janeiro, which was published in the journal *Applied Psychophysiology and Biofeedback* in 2016. Nineteen cyclists completed a stationary time trial that consisted of four laps of 9.9 (simulated) kilometers. Upon completing each lap, the cyclists reported their current rate of perceived exertion (RPE) on a 1–100 scale. Viana's team found that, across all subjects, perceived effort ratings increased linearly and peaked at 100 points at the end of the time trial. This pattern was so consistent that anyone with sufficient math skill who was told nothing about the time trial except what the subjects' perceived effort ratings were after the first two laps would have been able to accurately predict the total distance of the time trial.

Further evidence that perceived effort runs the show in pacing comes from studies involving the use of deceptive performance feedback during time trials. In one such study, experienced cyclists completed four simulated 10-mile time trials, receiving accurate performance feedback on one occasion, no feedback on a second, and inaccurate feedback (either 5 percent better or 5 percent worse than actual) on the other two. Despite these disparate informational environments, the cyclists completed all four time trials in about the same time, indicating that they relied on perceived effort rather than objective information to determine how fast they could really go.

In our age of technological hyperdependency, we are quick to assume that our devices are more reliable than our perceptions. The thing to understand about endurance performance is that perceptions don't just indicate our limits, they *are* our limits. When you feel you can't run any harder, you can't, and when you feel you can, you can—no matter what the numbers say.

Imagine telling a friend that you feel cold, only to hear your friend say, "No, you're not. It's 80 degrees." You'd probably look at her like she was crazy, and you'd be right to do so, because to feel cold is to be cold, regardless of the actual environmental temperature. It's the same with perception of effort. This perception decides how fast you can go, and no objective metric can be more "right" than this subjective feeling.

WHAT IT MEANS TO BE GOOD AT PACING

We are now in a position to say what it means to pace well. Perhaps the most definitive statement we can make in this regard is that every race should end with an all-out sprint to the finish line. We know this because we know that pacing is a matter of conscious decision-making, and to choose to do anything other than run all-out in the homestretch of a race is to voluntarily add a few avoidable seconds to your final time.

It is not humanly possible to sustain a maximal effort for longer than about 30 seconds, however. Studies have shown that when athletes reach a point where they feel they are working as hard as they can, they are within 30 seconds of stopping. In events lasting longer than 30 seconds, therefore, runners need to pace themselves in such a way that their perceived effort level stays below maximum until they are within 30 seconds of the finish line, at which point they can (and should) transition to a full sprint. Sprinting is relative, though. The more fatigued you are when you start a sprint, the slower that sprint will be compared to a sprint on fresh legs. Your closing kick at the end of a 100-mile race might not look like a sprint to an outside observer, but it can and should be a true maximal effort nonetheless.

Obviously, in a long-distance event, what happens before you're 30 seconds from the finish line matters a lot more than what happens within those final 30 seconds. The science of pacing suggests that you should run hard enough throughout the event that when you start your sprint, you're able to speed up only slightly due to accumulated fatigue. Remember, the objective of your pacing tactics is to get as close to your physical limit as you possibly can. This requires that you save something for the end of the race, but only just enough. The ability to speed up dramatically in the homestretch indicates you saved too much, whereas not saving enough will cause you to feel that you are running as hard as you can before you're within 30 seconds of the finish line, and because you can't run as hard as you can longer than 30 seconds on either fresh legs or tired legs, this miscalculation will cause you to slow down and lose time in the latter stages of the event (or even earlier if you really blow it). Optimal pacing, then, will cause your perceived effort level to rise at a steady rate that results in an almost seamless transition to your closing kick, a subtle shift from holding back a tiny bit to giving everything you've got that yields a modest increase in speed.

If this seems impossible to pull off, you're probably right. The description of optimal pacing I've just offered is an oversimplification. In the real world, no race performance looks exactly like this platonic ideal, although the best ones (like Kenenisa Bekele's 2019 Berlin Marathon performance) do resemble it quite closely. In fact, perfect pacing is not only unachievable in all likelihood, but it's also unknowable.

Simply stated, it is impossible to know for sure whether a particular race performance was paced optimally. Why? A few reasons. One is competition. Racing to win is different from racing for time. It often happens that the tactics a runner uses to get to the finish line first—such as the "sit and kick" approach"—result in a slower time than he might have achieved otherwise. Topography and other environmental conditions also complicate pacing. For example, the laws of physics dictate that, although it is not possible to run as fast uphill as on level ground, it is possible to sustain a higher intensity. Consequently, optimal pacing on a hilly race course looks a bit more erratic than optimal pacing in a flat race. Also, as any experienced runner can tell you, perceived effort does not increase with perfect predictability; there can be fluctuations, caused by who-knows-what, that defy this overall pattern. The best pacers know how to ease back just enough when they hit a rough patch in a race and how also to take advantage of a second wind.

Let's not get bogged down in such details, though. The main thing I want you to take away from this chapter is a clear understanding of what you're trying to achieve with pacing and what it means to run free by pacing well. Now let's talk about why you currently suck at pacing.

3

Why You Suck at Pacing

In 2016, Scottish anthropologist Michael Crawley relocated to Ethiopia, where he spent fifteen months learning about the country's elite running culture. A talented runner himself, Crawley did most of his fieldwork literally on the run, trying and very often failing to keep up with his subjects. But even when he couldn't keep up, things had a way of working out.

One day Crawley was running alone on a gravel road east of Addis Ababa, having once again lost contact with his training partners, when he was caught from behind by a stranger in Adidas racing flats who, instead of overtaking Crawley, offered to run with him. The Scotsman demurred, citing the need to take it easy, but the stranger wasn't having it and pressed Crawley to name his preferred pace, promising that whatever it was, he would make it happen.

"Four minutes per kilometer," Crawley conceded.

"Perfect," said the stranger, who was not wearing a watch.

"No GPS?" Crawley asked, dubious.

"It is in here," the stranger said, pointing to his temple.

Sure enough, the next kilometer was completed in four minutes flat. It was then that Crawley learned his companion was formerly a professional race "rabbit" who had twice paced his countryman Haile Gebrselassie to marathon world records in Berlin.

If every runner were capable of banging out a precise 4-minute kilometer on command, Crawley wouldn't have considered this story worth telling.

In fact, though, few runners possess the pacing chops to replicate the show put on by Gebrselassie's former wingman, which Crawley duly recounted in *Out of Thin Air: Running Wisdom and Magic from Above the Clouds in Ethiopia*. After reading the book I experienced a kind of counterpoint to Crawley's encounter that supplied me with further evidence (as if I needed it) that pacing masters are the exception, not the rule. It happened during a virtual running camp hosted by my friend Greg McMillan. On day two of the three-day affair, the campers completed a challenge that required them to run a mile at their individual lactate threshold pace without consulting their watch. Afterward we gathered online to share the results, and the results weren't pretty. One runner was off the mark by 40 seconds, while another confessed to peeking at her watch halfway through the challenge, powerless to resist the force of habit. Even the winner was off by several seconds.

All fun and games, though, right? Wrong. The pacing feat that Michael Crawley witnessed on a gravel road east of Addis Ababa wasn't just some frivolous party trick. Nor was the inability of Greg McMillan's campers to judge their pace accurately a matter of inconsequence for their training and racing. To the contrary, a runner who is able to run an exact 4-minute kilometer upon request is a runner who is also capable of executing better workouts and of realizing her full potential in races.

Good pacing is all about accuracy. To find your absolute limit in a race without exceeding it is to score a bull's-eye of sorts. It is only to be expected that the runners who succeed most fully in this effort are also, like Michael Crawley's pacing angel, really darn good at measuring things by feel when they run. But pacing skill is difficult to appreciate. A runner who is in the process of pacing brilliantly doesn't look any different from a runner who's in the process of pacing disastrously. Both just look like guys running. Pacing feats like Crawley's friend's four-flat kilometer demonstrate how good the best pacers really are—and not only when showing off for visiting ethnographers, but also in real competition.

I'm not suggesting you have to achieve uncanny exactitude in measuring your runs by feel to find your limit in races. I'm just trying to establish how far away most of us are from pacing mastery. For every retired race rabbit dropping four-flat kilometers on command, there are two dozen McMillan Running

Camp participants missing their one-mile time target by 40 seconds, give or take. To put it bluntly, the majority of runners suck at pacing. Odds are *you* suck at pacing. (Or did you pick up this book accidentally?) As to why pacing mastery is so rare, I see three main reasons, none of them insurmountable. But before we can surmount them, we must first name them.

REASON #1: PACING IS HARD!

Snowboarders who lack the ability to execute a triple cork don't beat themselves up for it. Why not? Because it's one of the most difficult snowboard tricks ever invented and only a handful of boarders on earth can pull it off. Watch a few clips of triple corks on YouTube and you will see how hard it looks. Pacing, on the other hand, doesn't look hard at all.

As they say, however, looks can be deceiving. A marathon, for example, is a race of roughly 55,000 steps. Completing a marathon in the least time possible requires that a runner execute every single one of those steps at a speed that contributes to this goal. The precision involved in optimal marathon pacing is about equal to that of the 2021 landing of NASA's automobile-sized Perseverance spacecraft on a 20-square-mile target located inside a crater on the planet Mars, some 250 million miles from Earth. Except NASA's engineers had mathematics and physics to go by, whereas runners must literally feel their way to this level of preciseness.

Neuroscientist Vincent Walsh of the Institute of Cognitive Neuroscience has argued that piloting the body through an endurance race is among the most difficult tasks the brain can perform, subjecting our most vital organ to the simultaneous demands of driving maximal levels of motor output, managing crisis-level discomfort, and handling the immense cognitive and perceptual challenge that pacing presents. We tend to think of sophisticated mental operations such as landing a spacecraft on Mars as requiring more brainpower than athletic challenges like running a 50K trail running event. But in fact the opposite is true, because an endurance race entails both mental work and physical work, and physical work *is* mental work. As science fiction writer Ted Chiang wrote in the novella "Understand," "It is a misconception to think that during evolution humans sacrificed physical skill in exchange for intelligence: wielding one's body is a mental activity."

It is a proven fact that cognitively demanding tasks, such as taking a math test, result in high levels of brain fatigue. Know what else is cognitively demanding? Pacing a running race.

Science has also demonstrated that sustained efforts of emotional regulation—things like trying to stay calm in stressful situations—produce high levels of brain fatigue. Have you ever done a running race? (Duh.) Then you can attest that chasing your limit is also a sustained effort to regulate emotion.

Research has shown as well that exhaustive physical work produces high levels of brain fatigue. Would you agree that "exhaustive physical exercise" is a good description of a running race? Thought so.

Finding your limit in a running race is like taking a math test, trying to keep calm in a stressful situation, and working to exhaustion all at the same time, taxing the soggy, electrified, three-pound organ that makes us who we are more severely than just about anything we experience in our everyday lives. That's hard!

REASON #2: EXPERIENCE MATTERS

Around the same time Michael Crawley was being paced through a long run in Ethiopia by Haile Gebrselassie's former marathon pacer, I was trying less successfully to pace my nephew Caleb through the High Street Hustle 1K Kids Run in Salem, Oregon. My brother Josh had asked me to run with his six-year-old while he accompanied Caleb's younger brother, Luca. Minutes before the start, I gave my young charge a brief strategy talk.

"Don't go out too fast," I cautioned. "All the other kids are going to take off at full speed and blow up. If you start a little slower, you'll pass them up at the end. Got it?"

The hint of impatience I picked up from Caleb's shrugging promise to heed my advice struck me as slightly ominous. Sure enough, when the horn blared, my nephew took off at a dead sprint, right along with everyone else. The fastest kid in his soccer league, Caleb shot ahead at a velocity that demanded a real effort on my part to match. Recognizing that, at this point, experience would probably be his best teacher, I kept a half step behind him as he pursued the leader, an eight-year-old dressed in a super cool lime-green racing kit with jagged black stripes.

Caleb's chickens came home to roost at the traffic cone marking the halfway point. His breathing became audible, his pace slowed, and he looked up at me two or three times with an uncertain expression. *This could get ugly*, I thought. And it did. Caleb's wheezing intensified to the point I feared he might have an asthma attack (even though he doesn't have asthma). He put up a brave fight, I must say, mustering two or three kamikaze surges before crossing the line second in a very respectable time of 4:42.

If you're smiling right now, it's because you've seen children, either yours or someone else's, endure the same ordeal—or because Caleb reminds you of yourself in your first race. Poor pacing, particularly the pacing error of starting too fast, is the signature first-time endurance racer's error, an almost universal rite of passage.

No human is born a pacing master. Sure, some runners have a greater knack for pacing than others do, but even the most naturally skilled pacers require plenty of practice to achieve true mastery. Through repetition, runners get better at comprehending abstract distances, develop a subtler sense of time, become more skilled at reading their perceptions, learn more effective ways of tuning their attentional focus, and gain a better feel for their physical and mental limits—all of which contribute to more effective pacing.

Research suggests that the last of these elements comes first—that new runners often develop a better feel for their limits before they get better at the cognitive elements of pacing. This was shown in a study performed by Australian researchers and published in *Pediatric Exercise Science* in 2013. Thirteen children between the ages of nine and eleven were asked to run an 800-meter time trial on three separate occasions. Because this was a novel task for the children, it was expected that their performance would improve across the three time trials through refinements in their pacing execution.

And improve they did—but not through better pacing. Rather, in all three time trials, the children started too fast, slowed down significantly, and then sped up again toward the end. The true reason for their improved performance was simply that *they tried harder*. The 800-meter race distance is notoriously painful. Having never before experienced this particular flavor of suffering, the children were undoubtedly alarmed by the sensations they felt in the first time trial and thus regulated their pace in such a way as to keep their discomfort from becoming intolerable. But there was nothing solid or impenetrable about this self-imposed limit. Therefore, in the second time trial, understanding at least tacitly that they could run a little faster if they were willing to suffer a little more by trying a little harder, they did. The new limit thus established was no less a matter of choice than the first, however, so in the final time trial the kids ran faster still at the cost of even greater discomfort.

Other studies indicate that athletes continue to home in on their true limit through subsequent stages of athletic development. In 2011, researchers at the University of Lille asked twenty-five competitive cyclists—including six semiprofessionals, fifteen regional-class racers, and four club-level athletes—to estimate how long they could sustain a power output equal to 90 percent of their individual maximal aerobic power. The results were striking: All four of the club-level athletes gave estimates that were way off the mark, whereas four of the six semipros predicted their exhaustion time with almost uncanny precision. The researchers concluded, "High-level athletes may be more consciously attuned to their bodies and their own effort sense as a result of greater exercise experience."

There's more to pacing skill development than these perceptual elements, though. No less important is the ability to calibrate perceptions against external reality. True pacing mastery requires not only that you have a good feel for your limits but also that you can measure a mile or a minute accurately without a GPS or a chronometer. This was shown in a study conducted by Spanish and Chilean researchers and published in *Motor Control* in 2020. Thirty-eight endurance runners and thirty-nine soccer players were asked to estimate elapsed time (i.e., how long they'd been going) during a bout of sustained running. Among the runners, who of course were accustomed to sustained running, the average error margin was 33 seconds, whereas the soccer players, who although plenty accustomed to running were not accustomed to sustained running, missed the mark by more than 2 minutes on average, validating the authors' hypothesis that "[t]emporal and spatial perception can be considered as a cognitive skill of endurance runners."

An even subtler aspect of pacing skill has to do with what runners (and other endurance athletes) pay attention to when racing. Pacing masters know when to tune in and when to tune out during competition—others not so much.

Proof of this comes from a study led by Manhal Boya of the University of Essex and published in *Medicine & Science in Sports & Exercise* in 2017. In this experiment, eye movements were tracked in a mixed group of novice and experienced cyclists while they completed a 10-mile time trial with access to visual feedback on speed, distance, power output, heart rate, cadence, and time. The results revealed a strong association between performance in the time trial and where the cyclists' eyes went while doing it. The faster-finishing experienced cyclists focused mainly on their speed ("How am I performing?") and paid little attention to any other metric besides distance, while the novices scattered their attention more broadly, with distance ("How long until I can stop?") getting the bulk of their eye time. The conclusion that Boya's team drew from these findings was straightforward: "Experienced cyclists are more selective and consistent in attention to feedback during [time trial] cycling."

Relax. You don't need to *figure out* how to be more "selective and consistent" in your "attention to feedback" during running. The whole idea is that all of these things—becoming more selective and consistent in attending to feedback; getting better at measuring time, distance, and speed with your brain; and improving your ability to perceive how hard you're working in relation to your limit—happen naturally as the miles pile up. You don't have to *make* these changes happen; you just need to *let* them happen by continuing to run. This is not to suggest you can't accelerate pacing skill development through various active measures; you can, and I will describe some of these measures in later chapters. It is only to say that, for the most part, the process is unconscious, requiring no less and no more than that you keep running.

Consider the marathon, a famously difficult pacing challenge. The vast majority of participants in any given marathon hit the wall, slowing down dramatically in the last few miles. But not all categories of runners are equally prone to bonking in marathons. In 2017, Swiss exercise physiologist Beat Knechtle teamed up with Pantelis Nikolaidis of the Exercise Physiology Laboratory in Attica, Greece, to analyze pace data from more than 300,000 participants in the New York City Marathon between 2006 and 2016. Among their key findings was that older runners paced themselves more evenly and slowed down less than younger runners with equal finish times, an indication that they had learned through experience how to avoid a late-race fade.

If you've ever doubted your ability to become a pacing master, take heart from the example of Laura, a masters runner I met through Facebook. Laura's first six marathons ended in major bonking episodes. When she signed up for marathon number seven—the 2018 Rehoboth Seashore Marathon—she was resolved on breaking the pattern. More than just resolved, though, Laura was ready. Her failure to maintain a steady pace in those first six marathons had given her the experience she needed to know how fast was too fast for her in a race of this distance, and also how she should be feeling at different points of a marathon if she was to avoid having to slow down near the end. "I was determined to break 5 hours," she told me afterwards via Facebook. "I took it on very deliberately. I wore a pace bracelet for a 4:55 finish. I stuck to the pace for the first 13 miles. My plan was to check in at miles 13, 16, 20, and 23. If I felt good, I would pick it up a notch. At each juncture, I felt great. By mile 16, I was passing people at regular intervals. At 23, I still felt good. I decided there was no way I would allow myself to finish feeling good, so I started to run hard enough to feel the pain." Having reached the halfway mark in 2:22:56, Laura "negative split" the second half and crossed the finish line in 4:42:47, a newly minted pacing master.

One thing about experiential learning is that it is aided by an early start, which in running is becoming less and less the norm. Among the several reasons runners aren't as good at pacing today as they were when my dad was doing marathons is that they're taking up the sport later in life. The typical marathoner during the first running boom was someone who ran competitively in high school and kept going, but nowadays runners like Laura—who ran on and off in her late twenties and thirties but only got serious in her forties—are far more typical. Still, examples like hers prove that any runner is capable of using experience to pace themselves ever more skillfully.

REASON #3: DEVICE DEPENDENCY

In July 2020, fitness device manufacturer Garmin fell victim to a ransomware attack that completely shut down the company's online services for several days. Runners and other athletes who relied on these services for uploading and downloading workout data had to make do without them during this period.

A disconcertingly large number of the affected athletes responded to the disruption by completely freaking out, many publicly. A Garmin user myself, I did not freak out, but I did appreciate the panic I observed on social media as a reminder of how dependent runners have become on their fitness devices.

Not that I needed reminding. As a coach, I see daily evidence of the stymieing effect sports watches are having on pacing skill development. Following are a few examples of device overdependence I've collected from athletes I've worked with. Not all of them are specific to pacing, but each is representative of a general relationship between athlete and device that holds the athlete back from achieving pacing mastery.

Example 1: Anything for the Score

Icy roads forced Sergio to go slower than normal in the run he'd downloaded to his device from an 80/20 training plan. As he neared the end of the run, Sergio glanced at his watch and discovered that, because of the slow pace, he was not going to achieve the predicted Training Stress Score (a proprietary metric that factors together workout intensity and duration). To avoid this perceived failure, Sergio extended the run by several minutes, stopping only when the forecasted TSS had been reached, believing that in so doing he had salvaged the original intention of the run. The problem with this logic was that it assumed Sergio's slower-than-normal pace indicated a lower-than-normal intensity when in fact the extra muscle work needed to remain upright made the effort harder, as he could plainly feel. Then, by extending the run, Sergio made it harder still—all because he trusted an esoteric mathematical projection more than he trusted his own perceptions or common sense.

Example 2: Slave to the Segment

Ryan, a mountain runner I coached for a couple of years, ran the first part of a long, uphill tempo effort much faster than he was supposed to, and he soon paid the price, practically crawling to the summit. When I asked him during our next weekly call what the hell had gotten into him, Ryan admitted that the first part of the climb was a Strava segment he wanted to claim. "Forgive me," I said, my voice dripping with sarcasm, "I didn't realize Strava was coaching you now."

Example 3: Data or It Didn't Happen

While vacationing in the Napa Valley with my wife one summer, I received an unexpected call from Bob, a triathlete I coached. The few such calls I'd gotten from Bob previously had brought bad news, so I was braced for another injury report when I answered. I needn't have worried. Evidently, Bob's power meter had died at the beginning of a ride, and he was now standing with his bike at the side of the road, wondering if he should go ahead and complete the workout sans data or push it back a day and try to get the device fixed in the meantime. Hearing this, I couldn't decide whether to laugh or cry. In what possible universe could a dead power meter be considered a reason to miss a workout?

Example 4: Virtual Reality Takes Over

Amir completed a set of speed intervals on his indoor bike. Minutes later my phone notified me that the workout had been uploaded. When I analyzed the data, I saw a massive spike in power at the start of each interval before Amir settled back into the correct wattage zone. Knowing the answer, I asked Amir what was behind those crazy spikes. Can you guess? Bingo! Noticing a lag between the time he started each interval and the time his bike's power meter caught up with the change in output, Amir had pedaled like mad in the first few seconds in a desperate effort to produce the desired number, then slowed down on discovering he'd overshot the target—not once but twelve times in a row. Amir's a smart guy. On some level, he knew his power meter was lying to him, giving him yesterday's news, so to speak. Yet he acted as though he believed the number on the computer was more real than what his body was doing.

Example 5: My Heart Rate Monitor Says I'm Dying!

Kevin posted a concern about his recent training on an online forum that I moderate. Lately, he explained, his heart rate had been a little higher than normal in relation to his pace, and the VO_2max estimates his watch fed him after each run had dipped slightly. A newer runner, Kevin was becoming discouraged and beginning to doubt the effectiveness of the 80/20 method he was following. Having seen this movie before, I asked him how he actually felt while running, and whether he would be noticing anything different if he ran without his watch. "Now that you ask," he replied, "I think I feel fine while running, maybe even good, but when my pace is right and my heart rate seems high, I feel down about it and frustrated during my run and also after." It was just as I had suspected: Kevin's supposed crisis of fitness was in fact a matter of perception, an emotional panic triggered by information that had various possible explanations, all of them more plausible than the one Kevin had assumed in defiance of how he was actually feeling and performing.

Example 6: Happy After the Fact

Suzanne was crestfallen at the end of her tempo run, having fallen short of the pace targets I'd given her. But later, when she reviewed her power data, Suzanne

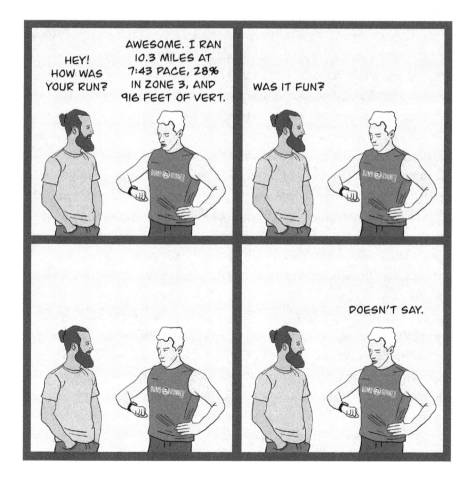

saw that, according to this other metric, she'd actually performed better than her device's estimation of her current fitness level. Windy conditions, I concluded, were the cause of the discrepancy between Suzanne's pace and power numbers. In any case, she was no longer disappointed. Mind you, nothing had changed about the run itself.

––––––––––

I could give you many more examples, but I trust I've made my point, which is that device overdependence is extremely pervasive among runners and manifests in myriad ways. Despite superficial differences, these several examples have one thing in common, which is a certain tension between what the runner's body and mind are saying and what the runner's device is saying. In matters of pacing, this tension takes the form of a disagreement between what feels right to the runner and the runner's interpretation of device data. Each such disagreement must be resolved one way or the other. It's a matter of who gets the final say, the runner or the device. Runners who are comfortable overruling their device are not overdependent and have a clear runway toward pacing mastery. Runners who are not comfortable overruling their device are overdependent and must gain the upper hand in their relationship with their device to become a pacing master.

Running devices aren't bad. They just aren't as capable of guiding runners to their limit as runners themselves are. That's because (as I mentioned in the preceding chapter) a runner's performance limit is not determined by anything a wearable device can measure. It is determined by subjective perceptions. If a runner lacks sufficient confidence in his feel for pacing and can't grant it the deciding vote in all pacing decisions, pacing mastery will elude the runner, at least for now.

It doesn't stop there, however. Running devices also rob runners of existing pacing ability through a phenomenon called cognitive offloading. Technologies such as running devices become extensions of the brain. We use them to offload cognitive tasks from our brains to external gadgets. The problem is that, when the brain stops performing a certain task that has been assumed by a gadget, the brain gets lazy and loses the ability to perform the task for itself. For example, research has shown that habitual reliance on GPS technology for navigation causes spatial memory to deteriorate and leads to measurable atrophy in the hippocampus, a part of the brain that's heavily involved in helping us find our way around. Running devices do something similar with respect to pacing skill. The more we lean on them in our pacing decisions, the worse we get at reading our perception of effort; measuring time, distance, and velocity by feel; and knowing our limit.

Too big to ignore, the problem of device overdependence has gotten the attention of scientists. In 2020, the journal *Psychology* published a study led by Pierluigi Diotaiuti of the University of Cassino and Southern Lazio in Italy. A group of 111 runners supplied information about their use of "sports trackers" and completed a questionnaire designed to assess device dependency, which was scored on the basis of how subjects answered questions such as, "If you could not have your device with you, would you still train?" The results indicated that most runners start off relying too much on their device. While some worked their way past their overdependence, others didn't.

In particular, runners who managed to escape device dependency tended to pass through clear stages in their use of sports trackers. The first stage was one of exploration and discovery—learning what their device could do, essentially. From there, runners moved into a consolidation phase, characterized by a more focused and purposeful use of key features. Then came the paring phase, marked by a rigorous selection of features that left runners attending only to data they deemed essential to goal achievement. The authors concluded that "more experienced runners . . . have shown that over time they have acquired a progressive mastery and internal control of their performance functions," and they were able to use "the sport trackers in a strictly instrumental way, for which there was no perception of dependence or submission."

Like I said: It's all about who has the final say, the runner or the watch. Runners who aren't comfortable overruling their device lack agency in their training, whereas those who get to the point where they trust themselves more than their watch gain a firm hand on the tiller of their running experience. Although this study did not look at specific consequences of device overdependence, I would bet my life savings that, as a group, the runners in this study who were least dependent were the best pacers.

A second noteworthy study on training device usage by runners was performed by scientists at the University of Twente and published in the journal

Sensors in 2021. Through a combination of interviews and diaries, twenty-two competitive recreational runners provided detailed information about how and why they used their training devices. A number of these runners had interesting things to say about the tension they experienced between their own opinions and those of their device concerning pacing matters. Their natural inclination was to turn over control to their device and run on autopilot, as it were. But what they discovered was that their gadgets weren't all that trustworthy in the area of pacing. To the extent they had offloaded pacing responsibility to their devices, however, the runners didn't trust themselves either, leaving them in an untenable, rudderless state. Some resolved the dilemma by tuning out their device data altogether.

"I feel horrible when seeing that I am not keeping up with a pace that I planned," one runner said, "so I start thinking if I should push myself harder on the next kilometer or punish myself by running slow. . . . I just avoid looking at it at all and check once I'm done because it influences me in the wrong way. . . . It's just not that helpful, is it?" You couldn't ask for a better description of what it feels like when you just can't figure out how to transform running devices from a crutch, which is what they start off as for most runners, into the tool they must become for pacing mastery to be achieved.

Experience alone does not guarantee that a runner will eventually get to the point where she trusts herself more than her device. Not all of the experienced runners included in the Pierluigi Diotaiuti study described earlier escaped device overdependence. For that matter, most of the examples of device overdependence I shared above involved experienced athletes. Why do some runners escape device overdependence and master pacing while others struggle? What do they have that the rest lack?

In a word: *self-regulation*. A hot topic in the fields of sports psychology and general psychology, self-regulation is a general capacity, shared by all living organisms, to manage their internal states and behaviors according to the demands of a situation, and it is critical to pacing skill. As we will see in the next chapter, runners must either have or acquire a strong capacity to self-regulate to learn from experience and overcome both device overdependence and the inherent difficulty of pacing to find their limit and run free.

4

Pacing as Self-Regulation

Humans are not the only organisms that pace themselves during physical activity. Animals of all kinds depend for their survival on the ability to distribute their energy efficiently when engaging in life-or-death acts like hunting, escape, and migration. Take cheetahs, for example. Zoologists have observed that wild cheetahs run significantly farther in hunts that end in a successful kill than in hunts that don't. This suggests cheetahs are able to accurately judge whether they are likely to catch their prey, and when they deem success unlikely, they give up the chase in order to avoid wasting energy. Interestingly, the longest unsuccessful chases are usually carried out by young cheetahs, an indication that they do not yet know their limits as well as the more seasoned hunters do.

From a scientific perspective, pacing is classified as a form of self-regulation, defined by the editors of the *Handbook of Biobehavioral Approaches to Self-Regulation* as "a process that allows organisms to guide their behavior in pursuit of their goals." As such, self-regulation is fundamentally predictive in nature. Goals lie in the future. Pursuing them effectively therefore requires that the self-regulating organism be able to anticipate the future with a certain degree of accuracy. This is as true for human distance runners as it is for hunting cheetahs. In distance races, as we've seen, runners continuously assess their effort level in relation to the remaining distance and adjust their pace in the hope of crossing the finish line just before they reach exhaustion. The crucial difference between this pacing task and a cheetah's hunting behavior is that the former requires the ability to comprehend abstract distances, which cheetahs lack. For better or worse, only humans can hunt invisible prey such as "10 kilometers" or "26.2 miles."

That which is uniquely possible for our species isn't necessarily easy for us, however. Much as young cheetahs struggle to know when a hunt is worth continuing and when to cut their losses, young and less experienced runners struggle to find their limit during competition. To date, most of the research tracking pacing skill development longitudinally has focused on types of endurance athletes other than runners, but we can be confident the findings apply to running. A 2015 study by British researchers found that fifteen-year-old competitive swimmers struggled to execute a basic pacing challenge (7 × 200 meters at incrementally increasing speeds), a failure that the authors attributed to both inexperience and cognitive immaturity. A separate study by German scientists reported that seventeen-year-old competitive swimmers performed much better in a comparable pacing challenge, indicating that two years of additional experience and maturation go a long way in adolescent swimmers aiming for pacing mastery.

Other research has shown that not all youth athletes improve equally in pacing skill over time. In 2017, the *International Journal of Sports Physiology and Performance* published the results of an ambitious five-year effort by Rikstje Wiersma and colleagues at the University of Groningen to track pacing skill development in a group of 104 youth speed skaters. Based on their recent competitive performances, the skaters were ranked initially as either elite, subelite, or nonelite. Interestingly, Wiersma's team found that, over the five-year study period, skaters in all three categories evolved pacing patterns that looked more and more like those of world-class adult speed skaters, but the elite-level skaters showed significantly more improvement in this area than those of lower rankings.

What to make of these findings? I think we can safely assume that, in general, the young skaters who were classified as elite at the outset of the study were more physically talented than their lower-ranked peers. But what these results seem to suggest is that something else besides physical talent—something that enabled these athletes to gain pacing skill more quickly—was part of what made them elite in the first place.

In a 2017 article titled "Pacing and Self-Regulation: Important Skills for Talent Development in Endurance Sport," Marije Elferink-Gemser of the University of Groningen and Florentina Hettinga of Northumbria University offered the following answer to the question just posed: "It seems that athletes who exhibit the greatest response to training, i.e., those who are most successful in improving their performance over time, are the ones who are eager to learn and train. They take responsibility for their own learning and training process, know which performance characteristics are important for them to develop, are highly motivated to improve and take action to do so. This goal-driven process is also described as self-regulation of learning and training, consisting of components of metacognition, motivation, and behavior. Self-regulation in general is the extent to which learners exert control over their own learning and training to master a specific task and to excel at it."

If this answer is correct, it means an athlete must already be good at self-regulation as it relates to learning from racing experience in order to get better at self-regulation as it relates to pacing individual races. The question then becomes: Where does a strong underlying capacity for self-regulation come from? If a runner needs to be adept at self-regulation not only to pace well today but also to learn to pace better tomorrow, what makes a runner (or any person) adept at self-regulation?

Psychologists have identified a number of mental traits that contribute to self-regulatory adeptness. Chief among them are body awareness, judgment, and toughness. There are others, but these three have the greatest relevance to the self-regulatory challenge of pacing a running event. Without exception, pacing masters are runners who possess all three traits in high degree. Some are born with a head start and require little experience to develop their innate gifts of body awareness, judgment, and toughness to the level needed for pacing mastery. Others are less naturally gifted in one or more of these areas and must bootstrap their way toward having what it takes to become a pacing master.

In its dependence on fundamental mental traits, pacing is different from a lot of other skills, like knitting, that are not rooted in self-regulation. Whereas knitting ability is limited by manual dexterity and little else, pacing goes much deeper, drawing upon core features of our psychology. If you really want to become a pacing master, therefore, it might not be enough for you to gather experience and practice pacing exercises. These things are valuable, but so are the key mental aptitudes that support pacing skill, and unless you already possess these traits at the level of a Kenenisa Bekele, you stand to benefit from cultivating them.

Fear not—I haven't forgotten that I am a running coach, not a life coach. In this chapter and the next, I will focus narrowly on ways to cultivate body awareness, judgment, and toughness within the domain of running. I'll leave it to you to decide how interested you are in growing more broadly in these areas. Personally, I find it quite appealing that the journey toward pacing mastery goes as deep as you want it to. I mean, what an opportunity! Why merely improve as a runner when you can improve as a runner *and* become a better version of yourself in the process?

BODY AWARENESS

Can you feel your body right now? I'll bet you can. Every organism with a nervous system has the ability to feel its body in various ways. The scientific term for this ability is *interoception*. To function effectively in the world, we must not only feel our bodies but also know what we're feeling and act appropriately in response to what we feel. The hollow sensation we get when our stomach is empty, for example, must be correctly interpreted as a signal of hunger that prompts us to eat.

Beyond survival, interoception and related perceptions such as proprioception (awareness of the body in space) are vital to mastering a wide variety of skills. Body awareness in musicians is one example that has received special attention from scientists. One study involving guitarists found that years of practice had led to adaptations in the brain's structure and function that made the organ far more receptive to subtle nuances in afferent feedback from the fingers. We all have brains and fingers, but master guitarists have brains and fingers that can feel stuff ours can't. It's the same with running. Through training, runners get better at using specific forms of body awareness, including perception of effort, to aid their running.

Psychology research has demonstrated a strong link between interoceptive sensitivity (which is most often assessed by having subjects estimate their pulse rate by feel) and overall self-regulatory ability (which is measured through standardized inventories that ask subjects to rate their level of agreement with statements like, "If I make a resolution to change something, I pay a lot of attention to how I'm doing"). It makes sense, if you think about it. Interoceptive sensitivity requires that the mind be good at listening to the body, while self-regulation requires that the mind be good at talking to the body. It is only to be expected that the better the mind gets at listening to the body, the better it gets at telling it what to do, and vice versa.

Pacing, of course, is deeply dependent on the mind's ability to listen to and control the body. As body awareness goes up, therefore, so does pacing skill. I wish I could cite a study proving this, but alas, the science in this area is rather thin. The best I've got is a 2007 study by German psychologists who looked at the relationship between interoceptive sensitivity and effort regulation in an exercise task. Thirty-four healthy subjects estimated their heart rate at rest and were then classified as either good heart-rate perceivers or poor heart-rate perceivers based on the results. Next, the subjects completed a self-paced, 15-minute exercise bout on stationary bikes. This wasn't a time trial—the subjects were instructed to choose any pace they liked—yet there were striking group differences between those with good body awareness and those with poor body awareness. Specifically, the latter group chose a higher relative intensity and covered more distance, yet they reported the same level of fatigue as the other group. The authors concluded that "good heartbeat perceivers show a more finely tuned behavioral self-regulation of physical load than poor heartbeat perceivers."

In the real world, good body awareness helps runners come closer to their limit in races, especially in challenging conditions such as hot weather. Humans cannot run long distances as quickly in hot environments as in cool environments because doing so would cause the core body temperature to increase to dangerous levels. But if we couldn't feel our bodies, we might try anyway, starting hot races at our normal speed and being forced to slow down or stop when we overheated. Thankfully, we can feel our bodies, so we instead reduce our pace very early in hot races, in reaction to sensed heat, when our core body temperature is still well below the danger zone. In fact, ingenious experiments involving radiant heat exposure have demonstrated that athletes pace themselves more conservatively even when it's just their skin that is warm and their core body temperature isn't affected at all.

A Master Class in Body-Aware Pacing

Not all runners have the level of body awareness needed to make the best pacing decisions. Even Olympians sometimes fail to make appropriate adjustments in adverse conditions. The 2004 Olympic Women's Marathon, for example, was held on a torrid summer evening in Athens, Greece. Despite a delayed start, the surface temperature was 95 degrees Fahrenheit when the racers bolted from the start line in Marathon, the ancient city that gave the event its name. Tucked away near the back of the throng was Deena Kastor of Team USA, heeding instructions she'd received from her husband, Andrew, two hours earlier in a cellphone call she'd placed to report on the conditions. "Just go slow," he'd said.

Not everyone did. The gold-medal favorite, Paula Radcliffe of Great Britain, surged to an early lead, with a wake of sweat-soaked contenders trailing behind, unwilling to let the world record holder get away despite the punishing heat. Kastor, meanwhile, ran as though the others didn't exist, seeking shade wherever possible, drinking twice as much as she normally would, and holding a pace that, although markedly slower than she'd run in breaking the American marathon record in London the year before, was the fastest she felt she could sustain all the way to the Olympic Stadium in Athens. Whether or not it was fast enough to put her on the medal stand remained to be seen.

At 5 kilometers, Kastor was in 28th place, but the inevitable attrition began soon afterward, with runners who hadn't bothered to adjust cracking one by one. By 10 kilometers, Kastor had moved up to 17th place, and at the halfway point only eleven runners remained in front of her. The only problem was that the leaders were *way* in front of her—nearly 2 minutes, and it seemed unlikely that nine or more of those eleven would also crack, thereby opening the door for the pint-size Californian to snag a podium slot. But then Kenya's Margaret Okayo blew up, followed by her countrywoman Alice Chelangat, and then Radcliffe herself, who was seated on a curb, sobbing, when Kastor passed her 3.8 miles from the finish line. With less than a mile to go, a wobbling Elfenesh Alemu of Ethiopia ceded 3rd place to Kastor, who powered home to claim the first Olympic marathon medal for an American woman since Joan Benoit won gold in Los Angeles in 1984.

Deena Kastor's performance in the 2004 Olympic Women's Marathon was a master class in pacing and an object lesson on the value of body awareness in the exercise of pacing skill. As it relates to running, this mental trait encompasses the full range of perceptions, beginning with perception of effort, which when properly attended to can "tell" a runner how hard to push at any given moment of a race or workout. A runner who has a high level of body awareness *just knows* whether to speed up or slow down or hold steady. Don't bother asking them to explain how. Body awareness, as it applies to pacing, is not unlike a singer's ability to match any pitch or an oenophile's ability to taste eight different flavors in a sip of wine. "Can't you hear that?" asks the singer. "Can't you taste that?" asks the wine connoisseur. And, "Didn't you know that pace was too fast?" Deena Kastor might have asked the twenty-five runners who were ahead of her at the 5K point and behind her at the finish.

As I suggested in the preceding chapter, one of the reasons so many runners can't feel their bodies as well as the likes of Deena Kastor is that they don't grow up running, as she did. And I believe our 21st-century lifestyle also deserves some blame, its many comforts and conveniences having in a very real sense divorced our minds from our bodies. Such comforts and conveniences remain largely lacking in rural Kenya and Ethiopia, and this reality—the greater physicality of life in these places—may be yet another contributor to the success of the distance runners produced there.

So, if you are not from these more active places, and you did not start running competitively in the 6th grade like Deena Kastor, how do you acquire the level of body attunement required to be a pacing master? I believe the most helpful things you can do are: 1) make perceived effort your primary intensity metric in your training, at least for a while; 2) practice specific forms of mindfulness that are intended to enhance interoceptive sensitivity; and 3) perform certain types of runs that challenge body awareness. I will show you how to do all of these things in later chapters.

JUDGMENT

Pacing is, from one perspective, a series of decisions. Throughout each race, runners decide—sometimes consciously, other times at a gut level—to speed up, slow down, or maintain. A well-paced race, therefore, is the result of a lot of good decisions and few or no bad ones, which is another way of saying it is the result of good judgment. In this respect, running is far from unique among self-regulatory tasks. Remember, self-regulation is all about guiding one's behavior in pursuit of goals, and from weight loss to earning a law degree, it's hard to think of a goal that doesn't require making decisions.

Human decision-making has been studied since as far back as Plato, but increasingly scientists are approaching the subject from a self-regulatory perspective. Among the leading researchers in this area is Jacob Hirsh, a psychologist at the University of Toronto. In his PhD thesis, which was submitted and approved in 2010, Hirsh observed, "Pitting long-term goals against short-term desires is among the most difficult tasks in human decision-making." It is also precisely the kind of decision-making runners must do in races, where the long-term goal of getting to the finish line as quickly as possible is pitted against short-term desires that include not wanting to experience the discomfort that attends striving for one's limit. According to Hirsh, making these types of decisions involves a competition between "'hot' reward-focused impulses and 'cool' cognitive control mechanisms." The more successful the decision-maker is in overriding impulses when they are inconsistent with long-term goals, the more likely it is that a favorable outcome will be achieved.

To do their job effectively in these situations, the "cool" cognitive control mechanisms Hirsh refers to must not only be strong enough to override impulses but also keen enough to correctly judge when an impulse threatens to lead the decision-maker astray. In other words, the job of the "cool" system entails performance monitoring and error detection as well as decision-making and decision enforcement.

A brain area called the anterior cingulate cortex (ACC) is known to play an important role in these processes. Researchers commonly use an instrument known as the Stroop test to measure how well this part of the brain performs. Subjects are shown a series of individual words, all of which are names of primary colors and each of which is presented in a primary-colored font. Sometimes the word and the font color match; other times they don't. The task of the test taker is to state the font color as quickly as possible, which is trickier than it sounds because one's instinct is to simply read the word. Performance is judged by the number of errors the subject makes and by how quickly her answers are given. In research versions of the Stroop test, including Hirsh's, brain scans are conducted throughout the process. What these images reveal (among other things) is that, when a subject realizes she has committed an error, the event is marked by an electrophysiological signal known as error-related negativity (ERN) in the ACC. The magnitude of the ERN is considered an indicator of the subject's ability to monitor their performance and to make performance-maximizing decisions, with larger magnitudes demonstrating greater ability in these areas.

As part of his thesis, Hirsh measured ERN magnitudes in a group of thirty-one college students as they completed a Stroop test. He then monitored the students' academic performance over the span of an entire school year, his expectation being that students with stronger cognitive control mechanisms as evidenced by greater ERN magnitudes would earn better grades. Hirsh explained as follows: "Self-regulatory processes are thought to play an important role in the maintenance of academic goals. . . . Conceptually, this is because student GPA reflects the composite of many decisions made across a long period of time. For instance, a student has to decide on any given evening whether to study for a class or visit some friends. The result of each of these micro-decisions (each one a self-regulatory challenge) is reflected in ultimate academic performance. . . . [S]elf-regulation reflects an improved ability to evaluate one's behaviour and engage the cool cognitive system whenever it is needed to sustain progress toward long-term goals." Sure enough, Hirsh found that students who exhibited stronger ERN signals during the Stroop test tended to get better grades.

The parallels between collegiate academic performance and running races are obvious. In much the same way a high GPA is the result of many small studying decisions, a well-executed race is the result of many small pacing decisions. We might therefore expect to see a link between Stroop test performance and running performance—and, sure enough, we do. In 2015, the journal *PLOS One* published a study in which scientists at the University of Padua had thirty runners complete a pair of tests similar to the Stroop test that were designed to assess response inhibition, or the ability of the cool cognitive control mechanisms to shut down hot reward-focused impulses. On the morning after these tests were completed, the runners participated in an 80 km ultramarathon, following which they were statistically separated into two groups: "faster runners" and "slower runners." Despite the fact that the decision-making tests were done at rest on a computer in street clothes and looked nothing at all like a running race, those who did well in one were found to have done better in the other also, evidence that better decision-making leads to better race execution.

The influence of judgment on pacing helps explain why female runners are generally better than male runners at pacing longer races, as was demonstrated in a 2021 study published in *Frontiers in Sports and Active Living*. Barry Smyth and Aonghus Lawlor at University College Dublin analyzed data from devices worn by more than 158,000 runners during a marathon and found that the average male runner lost 4.49 minutes compared to the average female runner as a result of starting too fast and losing steam. Other research has shown that men are generally more prone to risk-taking than women, and that women's brains exhibit greater activity in the cool, cognitive control centers of the brain when taking risks. Not all risks are the result of bad judgment, but aggressive starts to longer races are a bad judgment call that comes at a cost, to men especially. None of this means that male runners can't be as good as female runners at pacing longer races (as the example I'm about to share with you makes clear), but it does underscore the point that great pacing is impossible without good judgment.

What Good Pacing Judgment Looks Like

As I mentioned earlier, the mental trait we use to make good decisions is judgment. An example of what good judgment looks like when exercised in competition by a pacing master is Yuki Kawauchi's performance at the 2018 Boston Marathon. Yuki came to the race as a fan favorite but by no means a betting favorite to win. Nicknamed the "Citizen Runner," he worked a full-time job with the Japanese government and raced with legendary frequency. Indeed, he held the world record for the most sub-2:20 marathons run by a single athlete, but his PB of 2:08:14 was far slower than those of defending champion Geoffrey Kirui (2:06:27) and several others in the field. Nevertheless, Yuki himself believed he could win if he played his cards right.

His plan was to go hard from the gun, a risky strategy that became even riskier when a nasty spring storm struck the Boston area on race morning. Despite facing a 25 mph headwind, Yuki went ahead with his gamble, running the first mile alone in 4:37. But his intent was not to lead the race from wire to wire. To have any chance of winning, Yuki knew he needed to make the race as hard as possible for everyone, so he was far from disappointed when the other contenders chased him down, engulfing the mismatched agitator (green vest, gray hat, red arm warmers, white gloves, orange shoes) at 5 km. Yuki then made a smart tactical shift, tucking in behind the taller Kirui, gathering his energy as he awaited the inevitable slow-down. When it came, he surged again, refusing to let his competitors get comfortable. A pattern formed: Over the next 20 kilometers, Yuki yo-yoed between brash pacemaking and cagey slipstreaming, doing just enough to keep his companions miserable. But Kirui had plans of his own, and when a whittled lead pack hit the hallowed hills of Newton, he shared them, launching away so decisively that he was soon invisible, 90 seconds ahead of his nearest chaser.

Of the six runners caught flat-footed by the defending champion's attack, five had no choice in the matter—they were cooked. Only Yuki held back purposely, and it was his best decision in a day full of good decisions. Having scouted the second half of the racecourse on foot the day before (and the day before that), he felt Kirui's attack was too much too soon, and so he waited until he'd topped the dream-crushing Heartbreak Hill to give chase. By then, the defending champion was paying the price for his premature aggression. Yuki, half-blinded himself by fatigue and the elements, barely noticed passing the cratering Kenyan underneath the landmark Citgo sign en route to becoming the most unlikely Boston Marathon winner in recent memory.

Pundits credited Yuki's grit for his victory over faster rivals, but I believe his judgment was the decisive factor in this instance. Yuki had a smart plan, he was well prepared, and he executed his plan with the right mix of discipline and adaptability. There are five different modes in which judgment applies to pacing: planning, reactive tactical decisions, attentional focus, emotional self-regulation, and self-talk. Yuki handled all five of these modes masterfully before and during the 2018 Boston Marathon. Having set himself up for success by familiarizing himself with the course and committing to a fast start (planning), he ensured his success by pushing at the right times and not the wrong times (reactive tactical decisions), not getting discouraged when Kirui opened up a large lead (emotional self-regulation), ignoring everyone around him except the runners he judged most dangerous (attentional focus), and urging himself to finish with his best running in the final miles (self-talk).

Chances are you will never find yourself needing to practice good judgment in precisely the same ways Yuki did in order to win a future Boston Marathon, but you will need to handle the five modes of pacing-related decision-making with a similar degree of competence to achieve your best results, and I will show you how in the next chapter.

TOUGHNESS

The word "toughness" doesn't sound terribly scientific, but it is a recognized term in sports psychology. I find it interesting that every major running culture has a specific word for the same basic trait. In Finland they talk of *sisu*, which is usually translated as "spirit." The Ethiopian equivalent is *adegenna*, which means "dangerousness." Japanese runners strive for *ganbaru*, or "perseverance." And when American running legend Steve Prefontaine tossed around the word *guts*, his fellow anglophone runners knew exactly what he meant.

The many words for this one special quality that all great runners seem to possess tell us the phenomenon is both real and mysterious, definite yet difficult to define. Scholars of mental toughness agree. In a 2019 review paper, a group of authors led by Garry Kuan of Universiti Sains Malaysia observed, "Mental toughness appears to be multidimensional and most often associated with unshakable self-belief, the ability to rebound after failures (resilience), persistence or refusal to quit, coping effectively with adversity and pressure, and retaining concentration in the face of many potential distractions."

Sounds about right. But is mental toughness a single thing—as the umbrella term *toughness* suggests—or a bunch of related things, as suggested by the laundry list of qualities lumped together beneath this umbrella? Prevailing opinion among psychologists is that toughness is indeed a single, albeit multifaceted, thing. Among those who hold this view is Angela Duckworth, a researcher at the University of Pennsylvania who in 2016 coauthored a paper titled, "Grit: Sustained Self-Regulation in the Service of Superordinate Goals." In it, Duckworth and her collaborators argue that toughness (or grit) is essentially everything other than motivation that enables and compels people to give everything they've got to complete a task or achieve a goal. A task creates a focal point that ties together the various features of toughness (unshakable self-belief, persistence, etc.) into a single fuel that fires the effort. We have seen that achieving challenging goals requires self-regulation. But to do its job, the self-regulation process must have staying power, and it is toughness that supplies it.

The goal of finding your limit in a race is a terrific example of a task that requires sustained self-regulation, hence toughness. To my knowledge, there is no existing scientific research demonstrating a direct connection between toughness and pacing skill, but there is plenty of indirect evidence. In ultramarathons, for example, failure to finish (or DNF'ing) serves as a pretty good proxy for pacing skill—and for the toughness component of pacing skill, in particular. In a 2021 study, researchers at the University of Oviedo looked for correlations between various psychological variables and DNFs in a group of 356 participants in a mountain race. Of these runners, only 148 managed to complete the race. The strongest psychological predictors of a successful finish, according to the study's authors, were mental toughness and resilience (which overlaps with mental toughness). And not only that, but the toughest and most resilient runners among the non-quitters finished fastest.

Running is a painful sport, and as such it selects for tough individuals who aren't afraid of a little suffering. But within the running population, some athletes are willing and able to suffer more than others, and only those who are willing to suffer the most realize their full potential in races. Remember, running performance is ultimately limited by perception of effort and not by fitness.

A Lesson in Grit

Even at the elite level, races are sometimes won by the toughest runner, not the swiftest. The 2021 NCAA Men's Cross Country Championship is a good example. The fastest runner in that race was Iowa State's Wesley Kiptoo, who arrived in Stillwater, Oklahoma, as the man to beat, having just won the NCAA Indoor Track & Field Championships 5000m in a meet-record time of 13:23.77. Kiptoo's strategy in that standard-setting performance had been to start out murderously fast, demoralize the competition early, and cruise to victory, a scheme he executed to perfection, running the first 800 meters in 2:01—a pace that would have resulted in a world record had he sustained it—before taking his foot off the gas and coasting to the finish.

Everyone expected Kiptoo to replicate the same winning formula on the frost-browned Bermuda grass of the OU campus. No one, however, expected him to launch into the hilly 10K course at the same crazy tempo he'd started out at a few days before on a flat indoor track in a race of half the distance. But

Kiptoo did just that, running the first 1,000 meters in 2:31, or 4:03 per mile pace. This time, though, he had company.

Conner Mantz of Brigham Young University was known as a gamer, the sort of win-or-die-trying athlete who in every race either sets the pace or hangs on to the pacesetter till it kills him. Now here he was hanging on to Kiptoo, while I, like a true running geek, watched on my iPhone inside Taqueria Riverbank in Oakdale, California (where the carne asada burrito is excellent). I'd never seen either of these men compete before, but I'd seen enough running to know who was going to come out the worse. While Kiptoo looked cool, Mantz looked overheated—his brow furrowed, hands clenched, and stride ragged already, with more than five tough miles of running still ahead. I admire plucky running as much as anyone, but there's a difference between pluck and recklessness, and I knew it was only a matter of time before Mantz came unhitched, got swallowed up by the chase pack, and continued to drift backward, potentially costing BYU the team title.

I was wrong. But first I was right. Just beyond 2 kilometers, Kiptoo surged and Mantz came unhitched. He was quickly overtaken by smooth-striding Alex Masai of Hofstra University, on his way to catching the lone leader. Next came Florida State junior Adriaan Wildschutt, who elbowed past Mantz at the halfway point. It was getting hard to watch. Mantz ran like a stick pig, his eyes wild, limbs spastic. And yet, instead of being swallowed up, as the script demanded, the mustachioed mechanical engineer latched on to Wildschutt, who dragged him back into contact with Masai and Kiptoo at 6.2 kilometers.

The four men ran together for a while, Mantz looking by far the worst of the bunch. But as they say, looks can deceive. At 8.8 kilometers, Mantz pumped his arms and seemed to will himself ahead of the others, who could not respond. Grass grew between the new boss, clenching and straining out front, and his blindsided followers, gracefully fading behind, and by the end it wasn't even close. Mantz's bullish breaking of the finishing tape seemed like a retort, a middle finger raised at my failure to remember that a cross-country race ain't a beauty contest.

Performances like this one are deeply inspiring because they show us what is possible with a strong mind. At the same time, they are somewhat intimidating—because they show us what is possible with a strong mind! "What's your excuse?" they seem to ask. To watch a Conner Mantz compete is to be forced to admit that we have not yet found our limit in the toughness department. No runner can claim to have paced a race optimally unless he has left absolutely everything he had to give out on the course, and runners like Mantz are only too happy to remind us of this fact.

What does it take to give it 100 percent? I'll answer this question by asking another: Do you remember the lesson of *The Wizard of Oz*? In giving the Scarecrow a diploma, and the Tin Man a testimonial, and the Cowardly Lion a medal of courage, the Wizard pointed out that only a person who had a brain would want a brain, and that only a person who had a heart would want a heart, and, yes, that only a person who had courage (or toughness) would want it. If, as a runner, you earnestly desire to become tougher, you're already halfway there. The rest is just details. As American record holder Ryan Hall said, "The best way to become a mentally tough runner is to believe that you're a mentally tough runner."

I will explain more fully how to properly establish and pursue the goal of becoming a braver racer. Let's go there now.

5

The Mind of a Pacing Master

The best pacer I've ever run with is Ben Bruce, a now-retired professional runner and former member of the Flagstaff-based HOKA Northern Arizona Elite team. When I joined the group as an honorary member in the summer of 2017, I was far too slow to do anything other than easy runs with Ben and his fellow elites, but as luck would have it, Ben was injured that summer, and he was kind enough to pace me through a few key sessions while rehabbing what, at the time, he thought was a hip flexor strain but turned out to be a pelvic stress fracture.

The first of these sessions was a long progression run on Lake Mary Road, a hallowed proving ground for Flagstaff-based marathoners. As Ben ran alongside me, I was struck not only by his ability to nail the mile splits I gave him but also by how much thought he put into the process. Aware that I would be doing a lot more running, most of it alone, on the same highway in the coming weeks, Ben shared a litany of tips on how to stay on pace, noting tricky false flats, exposed stretches where headwinds were common, sharp descents that offered opportunities to bank time, and so forth.

In light of this experience, I wasn't the least bit surprised when Ben later transitioned into a coaching role with NAZ Elite that involved extensive pacing work. His *pièce de résistance* was a job leading Keira D'Amato to the seventh-fastest marathon time ever recorded by an American woman (2:22:56) at the 2020 Marathon Project in Chandler, Arizona. It was, I'll grant, a relatively straightforward pacing task, given the course's pancake-flat, multiloop layout, which facilitated a steady rhythm, but Ben made it look much easier than it was, shepherding Keira through 5 km splits of 17:02, 16:58, 17:02, 16:59, 16:55, 16:59, 16:55, and 16:56 before Keira dropped the hammer over the last 2.2 km as Ben peeled off.

If you're skeptical of the notion that some runners have an innate knack for pacing, good luck explaining Ben Bruce's mastery. Raised in San Diego, he got a relatively late start as a running specialist, competing in his first-ever track race as a college freshman after earning varsity letters in golf, soccer, and cross country during his high school years. Yet despite having less experience than his fellow Cal Poly Mustangs, Ben was by far the most reliable pacer on the team, in recognition of which the senior captains awarded him the pressure-laden honor of leading the crucial first repetition in workouts.

In Chapter 8, we'll talk about macro pacing, or pacing on a long time scale. Many if not most runners who are good at pacing individual runs are equally good at pacing their overall running career. Ben proved to be great at both, pacing himself to a professional running career that lasted nearly two decades, earning the distinction of being the only runner ever to qualify for and compete in sixteen straight USATF Outdoor Championships. And though he might not like my mentioning it, Ben is also the only runner ever to have finished tenth, ninth, eighth, seventh, sixth, fifth, fourth, third, and second—but never first—in national championship races.

The secret to Ben's pacing mastery is no secret. Like all pacing masters, Ben is a virtuosic self-regulator on the roads, trails, and track, endowed with all three of the key mental traits that pacing skill depends on. Body awareness? Check. Ben showed exceptional interoceptive sensitivity in leading his wife, Stephanie Bruce, through a bull's-eye 5:34 opening mile at the 2019 Chicago Marathon, where GPS data are famously unreliable, setting her up perfectly to record a personal-best marathon time of 2:27:47, averaging 5:38 per mile for the full distance. Judgment? Also check. Ben's remarkable judgment was expressed in a patient, methodical, even-keeled approach to training and development that enabled him to just keep getting better and better year after year. "I have always had a consistent mindset," he said in a 2012 interview for RunCoach. com. "Chipping away at times over the years has been the way that I have gotten to where I am as a runner today. . . . Not any one workout will make you a superstar, but a bunch of solid ones will make you super strong and ready to race." Toughness? Checkmate! I saw Ben's toughness firsthand in the summer of 2017, when he ran through the pain of an as-yet undiagnosed pelvic stress fracture that would have immobilized most runners.

As a coach, Ben shares my belief that you don't have to be a natural-born pacing master like him to become one. The preceding chapters served to define the mission: To master the skill of pacing, one must cultivate the capacity to self-regulate both during runs (exercising behavioral control in relation to the goal of finding one's limit) and between runs (exercising behavioral control in relation to the goal of learning to pace better). Cultivating the capacity to self-regulate, in turn, requires the development of body awareness, judgment, and toughness. The goal of this chapter is to offer practical instruction on how to do this. None of the methods you'll learn here qualifies as a quick fix, much less a "hack." The road to pacing mastery is long, but there's a prize at the end of it—the sublime joy of running free, which is to say, of knowing what you can do and then going out and doing it, every time.

LEARNING BODY AWARENESS

A distinction can be made between general body awareness and task-specific body awareness. General body awareness, or interoceptive sensitivity, is the broad capacity to feel one's body, which is measured through tests such as counting one's heartbeats by feel. Specific body awareness is the trained feel for certain body parts or movements that comes through skill development. The task-specific body awareness that, for example, a tightrope walker develops through training for his vocation is different from the body awareness that a runner develops through training for her sport. Whereas the tightrope walker learns a refined sense of balance, the runner hones a precise perception of effort, as well as other kinds of interoceptive sensitivity, including the kind Kenenisa Bekele used to keep his hamstring from shredding while fighting to remain in contention for victory in the 2019 Berlin Marathon.

As a runner, you're not interested in developing forms of body awareness that have little relevance to your sport. The time and energy you invest in improving your body awareness need to go toward measures that offer the greatest bene-fit to your running. Three of my favorites are body scanning, condition assess-ment, and time-limit estimation.

Body Scanning

Research has demonstrated that meditation and other forms of mindfulness (a state of receptive attention to the present moment) improve body awareness by modulating the insula, a brain region involved in interoception. Body scanning is a mindfulness practice that targets body awareness directly, and it can be done both during running and at rest.

RUNNING BODY SCAN

To scan your body while running, focus your attention on one small piece of your overall experience at a time, pausing long enough to notice everything there is to notice before moving on to the next piece. Your breathing is a good place to start. Don't try to control or change it; just notice it. Take some time to attend to your perception of effort. Try to pick up its nuances. Words such as "hard" and "easy" don't even begin to capture all that's going on with effort perception at any given moment. For example, the sort of hard effort you might experience when running slowly in a state of extreme fatigue is very different from the sort you might experience during the third lap of a one-mile track race.

Other aspects of the running experience you can focus on include soreness and other forms of discomfort in your musculoskeletal system, the rhythm of your arm and leg movements, specific parts of your body (even your toes!), tension in your face and shoulders, your perception of speed and movement through space, and the various interfaces between your body and the environment: contact between your feet and the ground, gravitational resistance, and the feeling of air brushing against your skin.

Runners are always aware of their body when running, of course, but conducting a formal body scan while running is as different from this default awareness as meditation is from daydreaming. The goal is not to scan your body continuously throughout every run—that would drive you nuts. Focusing too much on internal perceptions is actually harmful to performance, for reasons I will explain when we explore race pacing in Chapter 7. Just scan your body for a few minutes at a time when it crosses your mind to do so. Over time, you will develop a better sense of how to interpret and use what you're feeling to inform your pacing decisions.

BODY SCAN MEDITATION

If you practice meditation, adding body scan meditations to your routine can be a nice complement to running body scans. These can be done anytime—before a run, after a run, or whenever you normally meditate. Sit comfortably in a quiet environment and allow your attention to roam from one focal point to the next. Start by attending to the overall position of your body, then concentrate on where you are in space and how you're feeling generally (e.g., warm, calm, thirsty). Next, seek out areas of tension in your body, just noticing the feeling rather than trying to get rid of it, and then shift to your breathing. Now move your attention slowly from the top of your head to your face, neck, shoulders, chest and heart, arms, torso, stomach, bottom, upper legs, knees, lower legs, ankles, feet, and toes. Finally, do the whole thing in reverse, returning step by step to the overall position of your body.

If you're so inclined, include a heart rate estimation test in the occasional body scan meditation. To do this, you will need to wear a heart rate monitor with a timer. Take a few moments to focus your attention on the feeling of your heart muscle's contractions. Start the timer and begin to count the contractions. Continue for one minute, then stop the time and check your total against the current heart rate reading on your watch. See if you can improve your accuracy with repeated practice. You can be sure that any improvement you do achieve will translate into better interoceptive sensitivity when running, hence better pacing ability.

Condition Assessment

When I last spoke to Ben Bruce, I asked him how fast he thought he could run a 10K race at his present fitness level. Without hesitation, he answered, "Twenty-nine something." Mind you, Ben wasn't training for a 10K at the time. His recent running had lacked any real structure, consisting of a mix of pacing work for NAZ Elite members and easy runs done on a catch-as-catch-can basis. Yet he seemed quite confident in his prediction, and I have no doubt that his answer would have proved accurate had he given in to my arm-twisting and actually raced a 10K the next day.

Where does this kind of self-knowledge come from? I believe it comes largely from condition assessment, a practice whereby runners use each and every run they do to assess their present fitness level. This is something all runners—including those who struggle with pacing—do when circumstances demand it, such as when a runner who is training for a 10K race does a set of intervals targeting 10K race pace. But pacing masters like Ben conduct a form of condition assessment in all their runs, and the sheer volume of information generated through this habit is what makes the difference. Put another way, what makes a pacing master a pacing master is that he gets a feel for how fast he could race a 10K not just from a 10K-pace workout performed on relatively fresh legs but also from a random, short recovery run performed on tired legs the day after a hard workout.

To succeed in gleaning information about your fitness level from runs of various kinds you must properly contextualize what you're feeling. Let's return to the example of a run that comes the day after a hard workout. It's likely, of course, that you will feel tired and run slow in any such run. But it's possible that you will feel somewhat less tired and go somewhat faster than you have in recent runs performed in similar circumstances, and if you do, you may conclude from this information that your training is going well and you're getting fitter.

When conducting condition assessments, it's helpful to place today's run in an even broader context, comparing how you're feeling and performing—all things considered—against how you've felt and performed in similar circumstances in previous training cycles. Again, one such comparison won't tell you much, but routine comparisons of this type will aid you in setting goals and performance expectations for upcoming races.

Just be careful not to allow your condition assessments to become a source of anxiety. Approached with the wrong mindset, this practice could easily cause you to train in a state of perpetual worry about whether you are on track toward a goal, sort of like how weighing yourself too often or obsessively checking your stock portfolio can make you freak out needlessly. It's a matter of keeping perspective. If you complete a long run on a hot day after a poor night's sleep with thirteen weeks remaining before a marathon, when you're still relatively far from peak fitness, don't interpret the misery you experience in the late miles as proof that you're doomed to fail in your marathon. Conduct your condition assessments with a mindset of neutral curiosity. Account for everything—the heat, the lack of sleep, your modest fitness level, the thi

get fully race-ready—in assessing your condition, an

tral mindset in all of your condition assessments. Do

your race is tomorrow unless, in fact, your race is to

Theref

a pa

Time-Limit Estimation

Another simple exercise that you can perform routinely in the course of your normal training is time-limit estimation. This practice entails asking yourself how long you think you could sustain your present pace or, alternatively, selecting a pace you feel you could sustain for a specific amount of time. Like condition assessments, time-limit estimation, when used intentionally as a tool for learning body awareness, is nothing more than a broadened application of something all runners do automatically in races and time trials, during which every runner estimates, consciously or unconsciously, how long they can keep up their current pace.

Experience supplies runners with a general idea of how long it's going to take to complete a run, and at each point along the way we ask ourselves, explicitly or implicitly, *Can I hold this pace the rest of the way?* Experiments like the University of Lille study mentioned in Chapter 3 have shown that higher-performing endurance athletes are better at estimating how long they can sustain a given output, and that's why conscious time-limit estimation is a worthwhile pacing exercise.

Like condition assessments (and body scanning), this exercise is one you can sprinkle into your training in a playful way, employing it whenever the mood strikes you. Again, we're all accustomed to estimating our time limit in races and time trials, but what I'm advocating is conscious use of the same faculty in other situations—easy runs, long runs, tempo runs, whenever. It's just another way of making you more mindful of what your body's telling you about its abilities and limits.

Time-limit estimation is also useful as a way to regulate intensity in runs. Such estimates may either replace or supplement objective metrics used for the same purpose, such as pace. For example, most runners, regardless of fitness or ability, are able to sustain their VO_2max pace (or the slowest pace at which they achieve their maximal rate of oxygen consumption) for about six minutes.

The Mind of a Pacing Master

ore, you can target VO$_2$max intensity in an interval workout by selecting ce you feel you could sustain for six minutes.

Even when you do choose to use an objective measure as your primary intensity metric in a given run, estimated time limits have a role to play, helping you find the appropriate effort quickly, before your device has a chance to catch up to a shift in speed, and also helping you adjust your pace as you go based on factors like elevation change and fatigue. I'll have more to say on this subject in the next chapter.

CULTIVATING JUDGMENT

Similar to body awareness, judgment operates on two levels, general and task-specific. At both levels, judgment expresses itself through decisions. People who have general good judgment make good decisions in most areas of their lives. But we all know people who make good decisions within a special area of expertise while showing poor judgment in other areas. Every great athlete makes consistently good decisions within their sport, but not every great athlete also makes good decisions with money, in relationships, and elsewhere. To master the skill of pacing, you will need to cultivate better pacing judgment, and the way to do it is reasonably straightforward.

Research has shown that teaching athletes sport-specific decision-making skills improves their judgment on the field of play. A 2013 study conducted by Spanish researchers and published in *PLOS One* explored the effect of decision-making skills training in junior tennis players. Eleven players were separated into two groups, both of which played eighteen full matches that were videotaped. The first four matches were used to establish a baseline (so to speak) of decision-making competence.

After each of the next ten matches, the five members of the decision-making skills training group sat down to review tape of selected points with a coach, who asked the players to explain and critically evaluate their decisions in a guided manner. The six members of the control group received no such training. In the last four matches, decision-making competence was reassessed. On average, players in the decision-making skills training group were found to have improved their decision-making scores by 10 percent, whereas the players in the control group showed no improvement.

In my one-on-one work with runners, I've found that a similarly intentional approach to improving decision-making can improve pacing judgment. The tool I rely on most for this purpose is decision tracking, which is similar to the method used in the study just described. The key difference is that there's no video involved. It's just a mental performance review that can be done in the context of your training log. After each workout or run involving important pacing decisions, devote some space in your training log to assessing your decisions in the five areas that I first enumerated in Chapter 4: planning, emotional self-regulation, self-talk, tactical adjustments, and attentional focus.

Planning

Pacing decisions are made before a run even begins. This goes for both races and training runs, but for now let's focus on training. Among the decisions you'll need to put some thought into before training runs are where to run, what your pace and time targets will be, and who to run with. There's no need to fuss over such decisions ahead of less important workouts, but when there's a lot riding on a particular run, you'll want to set yourself up for success in every way possible (for example, find someone like Ben Bruce to run with you!).

The most common mistake runners make in setting workout pace targets is basing their decisions on their aspirations rather than on a realistic assessment of their current fitness. Aspirational workout goals inevitably lead to overreaching and frustration. Remember to always train as the athlete you are today, not as the athlete you hope to be on race day. Ensuring that your training consistently meets you where you are is precisely how you become the athlete you hope to be down the road.

Be sure to give yourself credit for good decisions as readily as you call yourself out for bad decisions. The researchers who conducted the tennis experiment I just described made a point (so to speak) of having subjects review as many situations in which they made the right decision as those in which they choose the wrong move. So, for example, if procrastination left you with no option other than to run in the heat of the afternoon, thereby putting out of reach a target pace that would have been manageable in the cool of the morning if you'd only gotten your lazy ass out of bed, take yourself to task. And if you nail a workout after turning down an invitation from a friend who always half-steps you and drags you out of your proper rhythm, pat yourself on the back. In either case, the process will improve future decisions.

Emotional Self-Regulation

Affect, or emotion, plays an important and underappreciated role in pacing. Remember, pacing is the art of finding your limit, and negative thoughts and feelings make it harder—impossible, really—to reach your true limit. This was shown in a fascinating study conducted by researchers at the University of Worcester and published in the *International Journal of Sports Physiology and Performance*. Fourteen runners completed 10K performance tests on two occasions—once alone and once in a group. On average, they ran 58 seconds faster in the group test, yet their pacing patterns were the same in both. The difference was that the runners experienced higher levels of positive affect in the group 10K. In other words, they ran closer to their limit with others because they were enjoying themselves more.

You, too, will perform better if you keep your emotions within the neutral-to-positive range and out of the negative zone in races and workouts. One way to do this is with positive self-talk, which is the subject of the next section. But before you can engage in positive self-talk, you sometimes need to stop negative thoughts. This entails mentally "catching" negative thoughts quickly and overriding them. For example, you might start thinking, "I hate how I'm feeling right now," during a workout, then realize you're thinking this and consciously put a stop to it. Doing so won't change the fact that you're suffering, but it will keep your mind from exacerbating the situation and dragging down your performance.

Acceptance is another technique that is proven to mitigate negative thoughts and feelings during exercise and to thereby enhance performance. This entails making peace, or being okay, with your discomfort. You're not trying to persuade yourself that you're not really uncomfortable—that doesn't work. Rather, you're accepting your discomfort as a necessary part of the task you're performing. You can't control how you feel when you're running, but you can control how you feel about how you feel, and acceptance is the most performance-enhancing feeling you can possibly have about exertional discomfort. Research has shown that consciously accepting discomfort increases endurance performance. It's mainly a matter of embracing the fact that discomfort is inextricably linked to the things that make finding your limit worthwhile for you. As the Nepalese elite ultrarunner (and former adolescent guerilla fighter) Mira Rai said in an interview for the Mindful Running podcast, "Running makes me happy. When you're happy doing whatever you do, pain becomes secondary."

Acceptance works best when it begins before running. You accept that the run is going to hurt and then, when it does, you accept that it does, which is always easier to do when the discomfort was anticipated. In a 2021 interview for *Athletics Weekly*, Norwegian elite middle-distance runner Jakob Ingebrigtsen described how he uses this anticipatory acceptance technique in racing: "I usually get really nervous, not only because of my expectations but it's also about the pain. . . . I don't enjoy being in pain. . . . If you are really well prepared and you do what you need to do going into that race, it's going to end up pretty good and you're not going to feel that much pain after all. But I know, going into my next race, I get really nervous [again] because of the pain. But I think that's my way of preparing myself physically and mentally for each race—to be nervous of the pain that's coming but also to be awake and focused on the task so I can run as fast as possible."

It's worth mentioning that Ingebrigtsen was only twenty years old when he spoke these words. You can be certain he wouldn't have accomplished all he had at such a young age (having already set numerous national and European records and won European and World Championships medals, he became the second-youngest athlete ever to win the Olympic men's 1500m event at the 2021 Summer Games in Tokyo) without such a strong capacity for emotional self-regulation. Take a cue from Jakob Ingebrigtsen and, as part of your post-run decision tracking, rate how well you regulated your emotions before and during it. Give yourself full credit for successful thought-stopping and acceptance, and admit where you fell short.

Self-Talk

I've always thought of "self-talk" as being a little corny. It brings to mind children's stories like *The Little Engine That Could* or Al Franken's Stuart Smalley sketch on *Saturday Night Live*—"I'm good enough, I'm smart enough, and doggone it, people like me!" Corny or not, though, self-talk impacts pacing, for better or worse. The kind of encouragement these fictional characters gave themselves is proven to enhance endurance performance. A study led by Samuele Marcora and published in *Medicine & Science in Sports & Exercise* in 2014 reported that training in positive self-talk improved performance in a high-intensity ride to exhaustion by 17 percent.

This type of "note to self" works best if it has personal significance or addresses a specific need. One-size-fits-all mantras like "I think I can" are better than nothing, but you'll get more mileage out of phrases that speak to your individual weaknesses and immediate challenges. For example, if you are prone to self-doubt, and you find such feelings bubbling up at a tough moment in a race or workout, you might choose to think, "Nothing to prove," to remind yourself that you are worthy, win or lose, and all that matters is trying your best. And if you find yourself beginning to overheat during a race and are concerned that dialing back your effort in response to this feeling will put your podium ambitions in jeopardy, you might choose to think, "It's hot for everyone, not just me."

Self-talk can also be used in more tactical ways to assist pacing. Two-time Olympian Ajeé Wilson of the United States liked to mentally divide her 800-meter races into two parts, the first 300 meters, which were all about positioning herself for the last 500 meters, and those painful last 500 meters, at the start of which she mentally recited the same script every time: *You're okay. You're comfortable. You're fine.*

Does every great half-miler use this same script? In other words, is Wilson's self-talk ritual necessary to optimize pacing in an 800-meter race? It is not. But tactical self-reminders of some kind, which can vary from runner to runner and from event to event, *are* required to find your limit, and they are equally helpful in workouts run below the limit. Over time, decision tracking can help you discover the particular internal messages that work best for you, just like Ajeé Wilson.

Tactical Adjustments

When Ben Bruce set his half-marathon personal best in Tempe, Arizona, in 2016, he faced a critical decision around 5 miles, where the lead pack he'd been running in broke apart as top contenders Scott Bauhs and Karim El Mabchour accelerated to a pace that felt a bit too quick for Ben. There were two options: go with the pacesetters anyway and risk hitting the wall, or avoid this risk by holding back and giving up on any chance of winning. He opted to roll the dice, and at 10 miles he found himself not only still in contention but feeling surprisingly strong, so he continued to press, chasing Bauhs all the way to the finish line for second place.

This is one example of the sort of tactical pacing decision runners are required to make all the time in workouts and, especially, in races. Over the course of a longer event like a half marathon, dozens of such decisions are made, and they range from whether to slow down and tuck behind a taller athlete while running into a headwind to whether to disregard a mile split that's so far off expectations as to suggest the possibility of measurement error.

It is beyond the scope of this book to offer comprehensive guidance on how to handle every conceivable type of tactical pacing decision you might encounter. Nor should you want such guidance. The goal is to become confident in your own ability to handle tactical decisions, not to have these decisions made for you!

In all seriousness, the tactical element of pacing is one of those things that's more learnable than teachable. By this I mean that intentional practice will take you a lot further than an encyclopedia of if-then instructions from me or any coach. For this reason, decision tracking is especially valuable in its application to tactical pacing decisions. It doesn't matter how bad your tactical decision-making is today. By reviewing and grading your pacing decisions routinely, you will become increasingly confident in the calls you make in the heat of the moment. But what if you lack the confidence to even distinguish good pacing decisions from bad ones? In this case, consider working with a coach to build a base of knowledge for your confidence to rest on.

Attentional Focus

The relevance of attentional focus to pacing is obvious. No runner has ever paced a race or hard workout optimally by daydreaming their way through it— at least not that I'm aware of.

There's an almost infinite variety of things you can focus your attention on when running, but all fall within a handful of broad categories. At the most general level, your attention can be focused either externally or internally. When focused externally, your attention can be directed toward task-relevant stimuli, such as a big puddle on the trail ahead that you'll want to avoid splashing through, or non-task-relevant stimuli, such as a squirrel scampering across a tree branch above you.

When focused inward, your attention may be directed toward thoughts, emotions, body sensations, physiological processes including breathing, and actions such as your step rate. These too may be either task-relevant (an example being assessing your thirst intensity) or non-task-relevant (like wondering how the Green Bay Packers are doing in their big showdown against the Chicago Bears). An internal attentional focus may also be metacognitive, meaning you're thinking about what you're thinking or feeling, an example of which is assessing whether your current perceived effort level is appropriate for the moment.

All of these examples of attentional focus may also be proactive or reactive in nature. Proactive attention entails choosing its object, as when you glance at your device to check the elapsed time, while reactive attention entails responding to a stimulus, often involuntarily, as when you hear your name shouted and glance to the right, where you see your cousin Sam cheering you on.

Research has shown that certain uses of attentional focus tend to aid performance while others tend to hinder it. Broadly speaking, non-task-relevant foci like thinking about what you're going to eat after the race are unhelpful. Sometimes you'll hear disappointed elite runners chastise themselves in post-race interviews for "losing focus." Seldom are such lapses as egregious as making mental shopping lists during competition, but virtually any distraction from the task at hand will negatively affect pacing and performance.

The mental trick known as chunking can be helpful in maintaining focus during longer events, where staying focused is especially challenging. Sport psychologist Noel Brick, whose research concentrates on how elite endurance athletes use their minds during training and competition, defines this trick as "mentally breaking down the distance to smaller segments." Thirty kilometers into a 50K ultramarathon, thinking about the finish line may be overwhelming, but thinking about reaching the next aid station is far less so.

The one circumstance in which dissociation, or intentionally not focusing on the task at hand, can be beneficial is when a runner's discomfort level verges on intolerable. There's a great example of helpful dissociation in novelist Haruki

Murakami's memoir, *What I Talk About When I Talk About Running*. While competing in his first ultramarathon, Murakami hit a rough patch during which he tried every psychological trick he could think of to keep running despite the overpowering desire he felt to stop. As a last-ditch measure, he tried telling himself, "I'm not a human. I'm a piece of machinery. I don't need to feel a thing. I just forge on ahead." To his amazement, this self-admittedly unhinged internal pep talk worked. Murakami did not literally turn into a machine, of course, nor did he actually cease to feel a thing, but somehow the very repetition of this thought enabled him to find a certain peace within his suffering and catch a second wind. "My muscles silently accepted this exhaustion now as a historical inevitability, an ineluctable outcome of the revolution," he writes. "I had been transformed into a being on autopilot, whose sole purpose was to rhythmically swing his arms back and forth, move his legs forward one step at a time." In this trance-like state, Murakami found himself easily passing the scores of runners who had passed him during his earlier rough patch. "It's weird, but at the end I hardly knew who I was or what I was doing," he reflects. "By then running had entered the realm of the metaphysical. First there came the action of running, and accompanying it there was this entity known as me. I run; therefore I am."

As I say, though, except in emergencies, dissociation tends to harm pacing and performance, as does thinking about or trying to control physiological processes such as breathing. Focusing on your movements can go either way. As a general rule, doing so is helpful when your attention is directed toward the interface between your body and the environment or on staying relaxed, whereas it's unhelpful when it's used to try to run "correctly" in some way. In a study that Noel Brick did on mental processes in elite runners during training and racing, self-reminders to relax were among the most commonly cited metacognitive strategies.

Different situations demand different attentional foci, and studies involving elite endurance athletes indicate that the highest performers are adept at selecting the right focus for each moment. If you think about it, this makes sense. In the early part of a marathon, for example, when you're feeling energized and excited, it might be best to pay extra attention to the current pace reading on your device as a way to prevent overzealous pacing, whereas in the late part of a marathon it's better to ignore your device completely in favor of feeling your way to the limit and urging yourself forward with positive self-talk.

At all times, though, your attention should roam. Whether you're 2,000 meters into a 10,000-meter track race or working your way through hill repetition number six in a set of ten, you'll get the best outcome if you shift your attention from one object to another within a limited set of perceptions, thoughts, and emotions. Pacing masters develop a natural rhythm in their attention cycling, a sort of attentional loop that moves from effort assessment to context-specific self-talk to pace checking and back to effort assessment (for example), with allowances for reacting to salient stimuli and changing the contents of the loop as the run unfolds.

The opposite of such tactical attentional roaming is fixation. Allowing your mind to fixate on something is almost always harmful to pacing and performance. Most often this occurs when a runner is experiencing a high level of discomfort, which then dominates their attention in the way that extreme pain does, but there are also many examples of runners fixating on less threatening elements of their experience such as negative thoughts ("I'm behind my goal pace") or emotions (such as disappointment) or even device data. At a press conference I attended after the 2010 Boston Marathon, a reporter asked Ryan Hall why he'd looked at his watch so frequently during the first mile of the race, which Hall had completed in 4:36. Hall explained that he had done it in an effort to keep himself in check, having run the same mile in an absurdly quick 4:29 in his Boston debut two years earlier. Not quite satisfied with this answer, the reporter informed Hall that he'd glanced at his watch no fewer than seventeen times in that first mile.

"I guess that is a bit excessive," Hall laughed.

So, hey, even the pros do it. But just as Ryan Hall (who, by the way, finished third that day in 2:08:40) admitted to fixating too much on his watch in the opening mile of the 2010 Boston Marathon, you, too, should confess your errors in attentional focus in your training log, while also noting what you did right. The following table presents the basic do's and don'ts of attentional focus during running, which you can use in making these assessments. Note that they apply only in races and workouts where your goal is to find or approach your limit. Different rules apply in easy runs, which we will talk about in the next chapter.

The Do's and Don'ts of Attentional Focus in Runs

DO	DON'T
Think helpful thoughts	Allow negative thoughts and emotions to go unchecked
Stay focused on task-relevant stimuli	Dissociate
Allow your main focus to be context-specific	Think about your breathing or other automated physiological processes
Relax	Try to control your form
Let your attention roam among a few key foci	Fixate on one thing

BUILDING TOUGHNESS

I am living proof that a runner doesn't have to be born tough to become tough. As a high school runner, my aversion to the pain of racing was so extreme that I committed unforgivable acts of cowardice such as faking injuries to escape it. When I got back into competitive running in my late twenties—having quit years before to escape the pain of racing once and for all—I was determined to exorcise the demons that sabotaged the first act of my running life, which meant embracing the suffering I'd previously shied away from. In this second act of my running life, the pain of racing was no longer just a vitiating part of the experience but the very point of it. I wanted not just to run well but to see myself as a tough person, and to this end I measured myself less by how quickly I ran than by how close I got to my absolute limit in the effort to run quickly.

Success didn't come overnight, but it did come. I will never forget the moment when, minutes before the start of Ironman Santa Rosa in 2019, I realized that I couldn't wait for the ten hours of strain and pain that lay ahead, and that I was as calm as I would have been before an easy 6-mile run on a random Tuesday. This state of mind could not have been more different from my state of mind before my first Ironman in 2002, when my last words (spoken to my brother Sean in response to the question, "How are you feeling?") before walking to the start line were, "I'm shitting my pants." It was a difference that made a difference, as the older but tougher version of me completed the Ironman distance 25 minutes faster than the younger but weaker version of me.

The keys to my transformation were *meaning* and *practice*. Becoming mentally tough was personally meaningful to me, so I worked hard at it. But meaning alone didn't suffice to get the job done. I needed to practice at being tough, again and again, for many years, gaining a bit of ground each time, like an actor overcoming stage fright not through hypnosis or some other instantaneous cure but by getting back on stage night after night.

According to science, mental toughness is 50 percent genetic, which means it is also 50 percent nongenetic, and for those of us who weren't born tough it is the desire to be tough that makes us tough. As the 18th-century English poet Horace Smith put it, "Courage is the fear of being thought a coward." Again, Steve Prefontaine's frequent use of the word "guts" comes to mind. In one famous instance, Pre said, "A lot of people run a race to see who is the fastest. I run to see who has the most guts." Regardless of how many or how few toughness genes you were blessed with, only by consciously prizing toughness—perhaps even making it the very point of your racing at certain times—will you fully realize your potential for toughness.

Again, though, it takes practice. One of the most consistent research findings in this area is that, for all of us, mental toughness requires repeated exposure to challenging and stressful situations that test our toughness. It was on the basis of this finding that exercise scientist Lee Crust and psychologist Peter Clough wrote in a 2011 article appearing in the *Journal of Sport Psychology in Action* that "to develop mental toughness, young athletes must be gradually exposed to, rather than shielded from, demanding situations in training and competition in order to learn how to cope." I would only add that the same holds true for adult athletes.

Other experts in the field of mental toughness have developed systematic methods for cultivating this trait in athletes. The two methods that I found especially helpful in building my own mental fitness and have applied successfully with athletes I coach are accountability cues and limit testers.

Accountability Cues

Codes, pledges, credos, mantras, and related tools can be used to hold oneself accountable to a certain standard of behavior. Through them, athletes and others transform vague intentions into explicit rules, and therein lies their power. In stressful situations, like when you're struggling in a race and beginning to doubt your ability to achieve your goal, it can be difficult to spontaneously come up with a thought or a snippet of self-talk that delivers just the right message to enable you to hang in there. Different from positive self-talk, accountability cues are more corrective in nature, and they obviate the problem of coming up with a way to stay on track by allowing you to fall back on prepared words that represent the athlete you want to be when the going gets tough.

It's no accident that many elite runners and other top athletes who are celebrated for their toughness have relied on accountability cues. For former marathon world record holder Paula Radcliffe, it was "No limits." For 2:20 marathoner Sara Hall, it's "The well is deep." And for legendary professional cyclist Jens Voigt, it was "Shut up, legs!" Such phrases counteract the panic reflex that threatens to control our thoughts and actions in difficult moments by providing an alternative reflex, not unlike how the mnemonic "Stop, drop, and roll" has saved the lives of many a person whose clothing's caught on fire.

The options are endless: "Never give up." "No excuses." "Be brave." The more personal your chosen accountability cues are—the more they come from the heart, in other words—the more effective they will be in holding you to the standard you've set for yourself. My mantra for my second Ironman was "Don't panic," a choice I based on the fact that I had hit the panic button more than once in my first Ironman and on the expectation that I would face the same temptation again. Sure enough, I did, but the words I had prepared in advance kept me from repeating the mistake I'd made seventeen years before.

With few exceptions, runners who truly, deeply want to be tough use accountability cues in hard workouts and races. All runners engage in some form of self-talk while running, but whereas in the minds of runners who struggle with pacing, self-talk often takes the form of an unstructured shouting match between base instincts and their best self, pacing masters put their best self in charge before the battle even begins through accountability cues.

Limit Testers

Training is more than a vehicle for building fitness. It is also a potential vehicle for building toughness. Each run you do should have a specific fitness-building purpose, but a select few workouts should be set aside for the special purpose of suffering for suffering's sake. I call these workouts limit testers.

A well-designed limit tester subjects the runner to intense suffering but is not so punishing that it does more harm than good physically. This balance can be achieved through workout formats that require you to run as hard as you can for short periods of time. There are two basic ways to run to your limit, both of which were first discussed in Chapter 2: closed loops and open loops. Closed-loop limit testers are runs or run segments with a definite endpoint that are intended to be reached at a maximum effort. Open-loop limit testers are runs that continue to the point of failure.

An example of a closed-loop limit tester is a set of six, one-mile repetitions where the first five are run at 10K pace and the last mile is completed as fast as possible. Another example is long accelerations, in which runners gradually accelerate from a jog to a full sprint over the course of several minutes. An example of an open-loop limit tester is the Prefontaine, where runners complete alternating 200m segments at one-mile race pace and one-mile race pace plus 10 seconds per 200m until they can no longer hold the required paces. All of these limit testers are included in the training plans at the back of this book and also in the library of workouts available at 8020endurance.com/on-pace-workouts.

Limit testers build toughness in two ways. First, they increase tolerance for the type of discomfort that is experienced in maximal running efforts. This was demonstrated in a 2017 study led by Thomas O'Leary of the UK Ministry of Defense, which found that subjects who completed either six weeks of moderate-intensity training or six weeks of painful high-intensity training experienced similar improvements in aerobic fitness, but the latter group showed significantly more improvement in an open-loop time-to-exhaustion test and a test of pain tolerance. The second way in which limit testers increase mental toughness is by enhancing self-efficacy. Runners who routinely make the choice to subject themselves to intense discomfort in workouts come to see themselves differently than those who do not. Specifically, they see themselves as being capable of *choosing* to hurt in pursuit of their running goals. As runners move toward pacing mastery, their running experience seems less like something that is happening to them and more like something they are making happen. Limit testers contribute to this wonderful feeling of running free.

6

Pacing in Training

Mastering pacing is not about learning how to run completely by feel, paying no attention to numbers. It's about finding your limit, which requires a fine calibration of subjective perceptions against objective measurements. Running free does not mean running like a wild horse, by intuition alone. It means knowing what you can do and then doing it. A pacing master is a runner who knows how she ought to be feeling 16.6 miles into a marathon, or 12 seconds into her seventh out of ten 60-second hill repetitions, or whatever. In other words, pacing masters aren't just good at reading their perceptions generally; they are good at reading their perceptions as they relate to distance, time, and speed. The best way to develop pacing skill, therefore, is to systematically train this specific ability.

In the preceding chapter we looked at ways you can develop the key mental traits that underlie pacing skill. Now it's time to shift our focus to the skill itself, discussing ways to improve pacing prowess by calibrating perceptions against measurements. There are three methods that I have found to be especially useful for this purpose: effort-based training, specific repetition, and special pacing challenges.

EFFORT-BASED TRAINING

Effort-based training is just what it sounds like: pacing yourself without the help of a device. It's okay to wear a watch for the purposes of recording data and knowing when to start and finish segments of a structured workout, but in an effort-based run you're not taking any pacing cues from your watch, relying instead on perceived effort to control your pace. The important thing—whether you choose to leave your device at home or set the display to show only non-pace-related data—is that you give yourself no option to cheat. When runners complain that they're just no good at pacing by feel, it's usually because they've never really tried, and they've never really tried because they can cheat as often as they like by glancing at their wrist. With effort-based training, cheating is not allowed, and it's amazing what a difference it makes for a lot of runners.

"I used to watch my heart rate like a hawk," wrote one such runner on the 80/20 forum after I persuaded him to give the method a try. "It got to where running wasn't fun. So I altogether stopped looking at anything other than time or distance on the easy runs, except for after the fact. Not even worrying about power, pace, or heart rate. Just doing whatever feels easy. It's been liberating not worrying about those things. It feels like the effort is always just right, and running is fun again."

How to Measure Your Effort

In 1982, Swedish psychologist Gunnar Borg wrote a scientific paper in which he claimed that perceived exertion (aka perceived effort) is "the single best indicator of physical strain." This claim was not well received initially by the exercise scientists whose turf was infringed upon by this claim, but today we know not only that Borg was right but also *why* he was right. As I explained in Chapter 2, it is now established science that perceived effort is the limiting factor in endurance performance. To feel you have reached your limit is to have reached your limit, plain and simple. Not every researcher who clings to the belief that heart rate or oxygen consumption or blood lactate or something else biological is the best indicator of physical strain has died off yet, but they are an endangered species.

Take blood lactate. Suppose you complete a standard, high-intensity run-to-exhaustion test, at the end of which your blood lactate and perceived effort levels are measured. You then go on a low-carb diet for two days and repeat the same test. When you quit this second run to exhaustion, your blood lactate level will be lower than it was the first time. That's because lactate production is affected by carbohydrate availability. But your perceived effort will be unchanged from the first test. Which of these two measures, then, is the more reliable indicator of your limit?

What distinguishes perceived effort from any physiological measure is that it's the only indicator of physical strain that comes straight from its true source, which is the brain. All conscious experiences, including perceived effort, emerge from brain activity. The hardest-working part of the brain during running is the premotor cortex, whose job is to make the body do what the mind wants it to. Brain imaging studies have shown that activity in the premotor cortex tracks closely with perceived effort ratings. This tells us that the primary determinant of how hard exercise feels at a given moment is how hard the brain is working to drive the muscles. Activity in the premotor cortex can be thought of as the brain giving the body a verbal command to move. When that voice is whispering, "move," running feels quite easy, and when it's screaming, "MOVE!" running feels extremely hard.

If the name Gunnar Borg rings a bell, by the way, it's because you're familiar with the Borg scale of perceived exertion, which went from 6 to 20 originally but has been modified (thankfully) to go from 1 to 10. And if Borg's name doesn't ring a bell, you might still be familiar with the three-letter sequence RPE, which stands for rate of perceived exertion and represents the Borg scale's units. Borg created the scale to serve as a way both to test his belief that effort perceptions are the best indicator of physical strain and to monitor and prescribe intensity. This work has continued beyond Borg's own lifetime, and what it has revealed is that runners have no trouble rating their current overall effort on a 1-to-10 scale, and that these ratings correlate well with measures of physiological intensity. It has all lead one researcher to conclude recently that "Borg's RPE seems to be an affordable, practical and valid tool for monitoring and prescribing exercise intensity, independent of gender, age, exercise modality, physical activity level and [cardiovascular disease] status."

There's only one problem. Scientific studies report average results, which tend to gloss over individual differences. And you'd best believe there are individual differences in perceived effort ratings. I remember reading that when American professional runner and 2:20 marathoner Jordan Hasay was returning to training from an injury, her orthopedist asked her to report her pain level on a 1–10 scale after each run, but he soon abandoned the practice in exasperation when it became clear that Hasay would never rate any pain above a 2. She could be attacked by a swarm of killer bees and still she'd report level 2 pain, maybe level 1. Similarly, I have observed that not every runner has the same idea of 2 RPE, or 5, or 7, or 10. Some attempt at standardizing the modified Borg scale must be made to ensure that all runners do more or less the same thing when asked to run for 15 minutes at an RPE of 6, or whatever.

The standardized version of the RPE scale that I use with runners was created through a simple process that involved translating the objective, physiological performance targets I normally use to prescribe intensity into perceived effort ratings. A small amount of fudging was required, but that's okay. There's no less fudging involved in intensity targets based on lab testing, which seldom yields the same results twice. So it's no big deal if your RPE marker for a particular physiological threshold is inexact. The only precision that is truly important in running is the ability to find your real limit in competition, and that's exactly what we're aiming toward here.

Physiological Anchors

The primary physiological anchor point of my perceived-effort scale (see Table 6.1) is the first ventilatory threshold (VT_1), which is associated with an RPE of 4. This threshold is important because most runners unwittingly do most of their supposed easy running slightly above it, whereas studies have shown that improvements in fitness and performance are greatest when the VT_1 is never exceeded in easy runs and other runs intended to target low intensity. The VT_1 also happens to correspond to the highest intensity at which a runner can speak comfortably. In your next easy run (when there's no one else around), try reciting a statement of approximately fifty syllables out loud. If you don't know what to say, I suggest the following:

I do not like them in a house.
I do not like them with a mouse.
I do not like them here or there.
I do not like them anywhere.
I do not like green eggs and ham.
I do not like them, Sam I am.

If you are able to do so comfortably, you are below the VT_1. If you can't, or if you're not sure, you're above it. Repeat this exercise periodically until you find the highest effort level at which you are still able to quote Dr. Seuss (or your preferred alternative) comfortably, and assign an RPE of 4 to it.

The other thresholds are less important with respect to their potential consequences on your fitness development but are nevertheless useful as they relate to the objective of getting runners on the same page. Your functional lactate threshold (LT) is the highest intensity you could sustain for about 60 minutes in a race. The RPE associated with this intensity is 6. Next comes critical velocity (CV), which is the highest speed at which your body can maintain a relatively stable metabolic state, and is sustainable for 20 to 30 minutes depending on the individual. That might seem like a large range, but in pace terms we're talking about a few seconds per mile, so minimal fudging is required to associate a one-size-fits-all RPE of 7 with CV. Finally, your maximal aerobic speed (MAS) is the lowest running speed at which your body will max out its capacity to utilize oxygen. In functional terms, this threshold is sustainable for 6 minutes, give or take, regardless of fitness level (though the velocity itself increases with fitness), and it gets an initial RPE of 8.

6.1 Standardized RPE-Based Intensity Scale

RPE	PHYSIOLOGICAL CORRELATE	TIME LIMIT
1	---	Indefinite
2	---	Indefinite
3	---	Indefinite
4	First Ventilatory Threshold (VT_1)	5:00:00
5	Steady State	2:00:00
6	Lactate Threshold (LT)	1:00:00
7	Critical Velocity (CV)	20:00–30:00
8	Maximal Aerobic Speed (MAS)	6:00
9	---	1:00–5:00
10	Maximal Velocity	0:30

Everything else is filler. Warm-ups, cooldowns, and active recoveries are tagged with an RPE of 3. This is an effort level you feel you could sustain almost indefinitely on fresh legs. Lower RPEs—specifically 1 and 2—are never targeted in training. Reserve them for walking the dog and climbing the stairs in your home. A 5 RPE correlates roughly with steady state pace, which is a pace you could sustain for two hours or perhaps a bit longer. A 10 RPE is a true maximal effort, which cannot be sustained longer than 30 seconds. This leaves RPE 9 to cover everything from a 1-minute max effort to a 5-minute max effort, approximately.

The Fine Print

Effort-based training involves a bit more than strict adherence to this ten-point scale. The first thing you need to understand if you're going to train effectively by perceived effort is that RPE increases over time at *any* fixed intensity. Heck, if you *walk* long enough your RPE will reach 10 eventually. Hence, the RPE assigned to any particular run segment is always an initial rating that serves to set the intensity and is expected to increase as you go, even as the physiological intensity remains constant. In other words, for prescriptive purposes, RPE assumes no prior fatigue. This means that, if I ask you to run 12 × 1:00 at RPE 9 with 2:00 active recoveries at RPE 3, your pace for both the intervals and the recoveries should stay the same throughout the workout even though, realistically, by the time you reach the tenth rep, you'd probably have to walk the recoveries to get your RPE down to 3, and when you start the next rep, your RPE will rise above 9 very quickly. It's just a matter of linking each RPE number to a specific pace or intensity that is fixed for the rest of the run.

More generally, there's room for interpretation, contextualization, and common sense in using the ten-point scale. For example, if I asked you to complete an interval set comprising 6 × 2:00 at RPE 8, and on another occasion I asked you to run 4 × 3:00 at RPE 8, you can and should exploit the fact that this RPE value, like the others in the scale, represents a narrow range, not a point, and run the longer intervals slightly slower than the shorter ones.

Effort-based training does not require you to completely tune out objective performance metrics (i.e., pace and run power). For the most part, you should completely ignore such metrics during RPE-guided runs, but it's okay and even advisable oftentimes to look at your pace and/or power data afterward. This can help you assess your pacing performance and document your progress toward pacing mastery. I'll give you a specific example of how to conduct this sort of post hoc analysis when I discuss long accelerations later in the chapter.

Finally, although it is possible to train effectively for races with RPE-based runs exclusively, I don't believe it's the most effective way to develop pacing skill. There's something to be said for training by pace or power in select workouts where the aim is to exercise precise control over pace. Indeed, such workouts do more than any others to calibrate subjective effort perception to objective reality. And when you feel you've achieved a sufficient level of pacing mastery, you can go back to using pace- or power-based training generally. The only run type that should always be done by perceived effort, in my view, is easy runs. This is because easy runs account for the bulk of any sensible runner's training time, and allowing your pace to fluctuate from day to day based on how you feel is a simple way to fine-tune your training load as you go. Affording yourself this latitude will help you avoid having to make the bigger adjustments to your plan that often result when runners don't listen to their body.

SPECIFIC REPETITION

The training style of Japan's elite runners is rather monotonous by the standards of some runners from other places. Pro runners everywhere run a lot, but the Japanese tend to run more than their counterparts in the rest of the world. Australian runner Melissa Duncan wasn't aware of this when she joined the Tokyo-based Shiseido Running Club in 2019, and she got a rude awakening in her first team meeting, where she learned that she and her new teammates would be running three times the next day—and the day after that, and the day after that; up to 200 km (160 miles) per week all told.

In addition to running a lot, Japanese elite runners have a predilection for loop courses. Boston Marathon winner Toshihiko Seko took this approach to an extreme in his 1980s heyday, doing most of his runs—including long runs of up to 40 km—around a 1.3-km loop. That was forty years ago, but a milder form of the practice remains common today. Japan's top runners tend to cycle through a limited variety of workouts over and over, as the world was reminded when Hitomi Niiya's training log was posted online after she set a national record of 1:06:38 in the 2020 Houston Half Marathon. Those who took the time to scroll through the schedule saw a small handful of workout types, most notably 400-meter and 1000-meter intervals, repeated again and again. A few workouts of other types (hill repetitions, steady state runs) are mixed in there, but not many.

Japanese-born running coach Nobby Hashizume once explained to me that the emphasis on repetition in the training of his native country's elite runners comes from the predominance of Ekidens (team relay road races) in their running culture. Tactical head-to-head racing plays a very small role in these competitions, while steady solo pacing plays a very large role, for which a highly repetitive style of training serves as excellent preparation. It stands to reason. When you do certain types of workouts repeatedly, you get to know them intimately, becoming sensitive to ever-finer details of the experience, which enables you to execute the pacing element of the workout with ever-increasing confidence and competence. What's more, this newfound pacing efficacy is to some extent generalizable to the rest of your running. It's sort of like how taking a deep dive into a certain musical artist makes you better at listening to all music.

Additional benefits come from comparing your performance in often-repeated workouts against your performance in races. Over time, these workouts become benchmarks that enable you to set appropriate goals and realistic expectations for races. It doesn't particularly matter which specific workouts you use for this purpose. All that matters is that you do enough of them in the lead-up to a race of a given distance to know how your performance in them correlates to race performance. You're simply doing the workouts, noting your times, racing, and then comparing after the fact, so that the same workouts have predictive value when you do them in the future. In the case of Hitomi Niiya, what she did in bread-and-butter workouts like 400-meter and 1000-meter repeats told her what she could do in her half marathon, but both the workouts and the race distance could have been different and her use of specific repetition would have had the same effect.

Simplicity is a virtue in such runs. A very basic workout structure facilitates both the process of familiarization and apples-to-apples comparisons between runs of the same type. So much has been written and said about training for running over the decades that those of us who write and speak publicly on the topic feel a certain pressure to create novelty. ("Here's an exotic workout you've never seen before!") An unintended consequence of such novelty bias is that it causes runners to lose sight of the value of straightforward workouts such as 12 × 300 meters at 3000-meter race effort.

Naturally, the workouts you choose to repeat most regularly need to have some relevance to the race you're training for in terms of their fitness benefits. A 4-hour long run is not the best choice for specific repetition if you're training for a 1500-meter track race, nor is a set of 100-meter sprints the ideal bread-and-butter workout to use in preparing for a 100-mile trail ultramarathon. The specific pace you target in such workouts should at least fall within shouting distance of race pace. You need not—and in fact should not—limit yourself to just one workout type, though. You'll get that much more out of your use of specific repetition if, like Niiya, you choose at least a couple of workout types, perhaps one targeting an intensity that's faster than race pace for your upcoming event and another targeting an intensity that's about equal to or slightly slower than race pace.

Also, the workouts you use for the purpose of specific repetition should not be identical each time you do them. Instead they should gradually become more challenging so that they keep pushing your fitness level upward. For example, you might start a sequence with 4 × 4:00 at critical velocity, advance to 5 × 4:00 the next time, and add a sixth rep in the third and final workout of the sequence. Note that all of the *On Pace* training plans presented in chapters 9 through 12 include sequences of bread-and-butter workouts chosen in accordance with the principle of specific repetition.

SPECIAL PACING CHALLENGES

Picture a contest for runners that has the following design: Each contestant stands alone with a "guide" at the start line of a half marathon. The guide goes first, beginning to make her way through the course at a steady pace that is unspecified except that the contestant she's partnered with knows it's slower than his own half-marathon race pace. The moment the guide reaches the course's first turn and disappears from sight, the contestant is allowed to start.

His goal is to catch the guide as close to the finish line as possible. Hence, the challenge the contestant is faced with is judging the guide's pace in the first 30 or 60 seconds she's visible, considering the distance to be covered, and choosing a pace that's just enough faster than the guide's to close the gap over precisely 13.11

miles. The wrinkle is that the contestant's performance is judged not only by how close to the finish line the catch occurs but also by how even his 1 km split times are throughout the chase, so contestants can't just game the system by closing the distance as quickly as possible and then shadowing the guide until the very end.

It's a wacky format, yet straightforward enough to function as a pure test of pacing skill. If 100 different contestants were to complete the challenge on five separate occasions on different courses and with a new guide each time, some would consistently achieve top scores while others would perform relatively poorly with equal consistency. And you can bet that the top runners would be the same runners who succeeded best in finding their limit in normal races, because when you're good at pacing, you're good at pacing. If you're adept at pacing routine workouts and normal races, you're likely to be adept (at least in relation to other runners) at executing novel tests of pacing ability, and vice versa.

In the previous section I made an analogy between developing pacing skill and cultivating an ear for music. My point was that repeated exposure to any particular kind of experience leads to more nuanced perceptions of it, which in turn lead to greater control. But there's just as much to be said for throwing curveballs at perception. In reality, no runner ever truly runs the same race or workout twice. In small ways, at least, each running experience is unique, and for this reason it takes a certain kind of mental agility to pace well with consistency. Special pacing challenges are designed to improve this aspect of pacing skill.

I must confess that I quite like the half-marathon tracking game I came up with, but it's not terribly practical. Fortunately, there are plenty of other special pacing challenges that can be done anywhere at any time without outside help while also conferring the fitness benefits one seeks in regular workouts. Following are short descriptions of a handful of such formats I've collected and invented over the years, all of which are included in the training plans presented in chapters 9 through 12. Feel free to create your own special pacing challenges—the options are endless, and the whole idea is to keep challenging your pacing skill with the unfamiliar.

Precision Splitting

These workouts develop your ability to hit the same time—down to the hundredth of a second, if possible—in each interval of a set such as 8 × 400m or

6 × 800m. There are two ways to go about it. One is to pick an appropriate target time before the workout and aim to nail it perfectly from start to finish. The other option is to run the first interval by feel, capture your time, and then try to hit the same time in every subsequent rep.

Obviously, this is not a challenge that works for time-based intervals, and I do prefer time-based intervals generally because they are one-size-fits-all. A set of 2-minute intervals at maximal aerobic speed is equally challenging for fast and slow runners because both are able to sustain this speed for about 6 minutes straight. But a set of 600m intervals at MAS is significantly more challenging for slower runners because it takes them longer to cover that distance, so they're coming closer to their limit in each interval. To get a pacing challenge similar to that of precision intervals in a time-based workout, try stretch intervals instead.

Stretch Intervals

This pacing challenge is made up of intervals of a uniform duration in which you aim to cover slightly more distance each time. For example, you might run 10 × 30 seconds uphill, completing the last rep at maximal effort and each preceding rep just a hair slower. The challenge here is to run the first rep at a high effort level that leaves just enough space for nine subsequent increases in speed. To execute this type of workout properly, you will need some way of marking the endpoint of each interval. I like to use brightly colored socks, dropping one at the finish of the first rep, dropping the other at the end of the second rep, retrieving the first on my way back to the starting point for interval number three, and so forth.

Stretch intervals improve pacing skill by challenging you to perceive tiny differences in speed and effort and to regulate your speed and effort with a higher degree of precision than you are accustomed to doing. Most runners find stretch intervals difficult both physically and mentally, yet also fun.

Fast-Finish Long Runs

There's a rule I sometimes impose on runners who have a tendency to fade toward the end of long runs. It's called the fastest-mile-last rule, and it works just the way it sounds: The runner is required to complete the last mile (or kilometer) of the run faster than any preceding mile. It's a simple way to encourage runners to be more mindful in their pacing from the outset, making sure they save enough energy to speed up in the homestretch. A majority of the training plans at the back of this book feature time-based long runs with a 5-minute fast finish, but it's the same idea and offers the same benefit.

Mind you, a perfectly executed fast finish is not an all-out effort that leaves you dry heaving at the foot of your driveway but a gentle push resulting in a split time that's a few ticks quicker than the next quickest segment of the run. Practicing this method habitually will train your mind to think ahead in all of your runs, including races, as pacing masters do.

Long Accelerations

Go out and run for 3 minutes, 6 minutes, or 11 minutes, accelerating continuously the entire time without consulting your watch. This is theoretically doable, as acceleration is something every runner can feel. In fact, accelerating continuously for much shorter periods—say, 10 to 20 seconds—is quite easy. But drawing out a continuous acceleration over several minutes demands a high degree of body attunement and nuanced pace control, and that's what makes long accelerations a terrific special pacing challenge.

In the preceding chapter, long accelerations were presented as a tool for building toughness. And they are that. But they're even more mentally taxing than they are physically challenging, as any runner who's done them can attest. The most common mistake made in executing long accelerations is speeding up too quickly, which results in an "oh, shit" moment when the runner realizes that, with time still on the clock, he's run out of gears. I call this pacing yourself into a corner. The limit comes more suddenly than most first-timers anticipate. So don't think about accelerating, per se. That's too black-and-white. Think about *accelerating as slowly as possible*—so slowly that it's hard to tell sometimes whether you're truly speeding up or you're making the second-most common error in executing long accelerations, which is plateauing in pace or even slowing down a bit at various points along the way.

Although you are forbidden to monitor your pace when doing a long acceleration, you should record your workout data so you can look at it later and judge your performance. Focus on the pace curve. It should be gently upward-sloping from end to end. The likelihood of this happening will be greater if you run your accelerations on a flat route. If you run with a power meter, an undulating route will serve the purpose. In this case, your power curve will give you a better indication than pace of how you performed.

Relaxed Time Trial

Here's how to do a relaxed time trial: Warm up and then run 5 km or 10 km at a 95 percent effort, aiming to cover the distance 5 percent slower than you would in a race. I started doing relaxed time trials many years ago because they seemed like a good way to sharpen up, build confidence, and dial in my time goal for an upcoming race of the same distance, but I've since come to appreciate relaxed time trials as a special pacing challenge.

The ideal time to do a relaxed time trial is about two weeks before a race of the same distance. Your performance is judged by the time delta between the two. If it's exactly 5 percent you get a lollipop. I've done enough relaxed time trials that I've gotten quite good at them. In my last one, I covered 10 km in 35:08. A couple of weeks later, I ran a 10 km virtual race (this was during the COVID-19 pandemic, so there were no real races to run) in 33:25, which is 4.9 percent faster!

The 5K and 10K distances work best for relaxed time trials because they are long enough to constitute workouts unto themselves but not so long as to leave you worn out and beat up for two or three days afterward. I myself have actually done full marathons as relaxed time trials, but my lawyers are telling me to tell you not to try this at home.

Progression Fartleks

Runners have a natural tendency to run shorter workout segments faster, regardless of instructions. For example, if I asked a runner to run 50 × 20 seconds at half-marathon effort with 40 seconds of easy running between surges, there's about a 95 percent chance the runner would complete the first few "on" efforts way too fast, reflexively tuning her pace to the duration, and pay for it later in the workout.

Progression fartleks are a special pacing challenge that require runners to override their natural tendency to tailor their effort to duration. I learned about them from Jay Johnson, a veteran coach who provides online resources and organizes camps and clinics for high school runners and their coaches. What makes progression fartlek runs different from and more difficult to pace than other fartleks is that the "on" segments get both longer and faster as you go. The hardest version of this workout type consists of eight on/off pairs with the following durations: 3:00/1:00, 3:00/1:00, 4:00/1:00, 4:00/1:00, 5:00/1:00, 5:00/1:00, 6:00/1:00, 6:00/1:00. The whole sequence must be done by perceived effort, without reference to pace or power. Aim for an RPE of 4 to 5 in the 3-minute segments, 5 to 6 in the 4-minute segments, 6 to 7 in the 5-minute segments, and 7 to 8 in the 6-minute segments. The 1-minute "off" segments are to be run at your normal recovery pace.

The most common error in executing progression fartleks, as with long accelerations, is starting too fast and pacing yourself into a corner before the end. Bear in mind that the "on" segments total up to 36 minutes, while the "off" segments are short and total up to just 8 minutes, so if you start the first 3-minute segment at your 10K race pace, you're in for a world of hurt later on. Be sure to record your workout data so you can analyze it later to see how you did with your pacing. Perfect execution is defined as running each pair of "on" efforts at a faster pace or higher average power than the preceding pair and finishing the final "on" segment at an RPE of 8.

DON'T FORGET TO HAVE FUN!

The biggest misstep that I made when I started to teach pacing skill to runners in a programmatic way was unintentionally making some of them feel like every run was a test of some kind. That's no fun, and it had a negative effect on the overall motivation and enjoyment levels of some.

We must never allow our pacing work to spoil the fun of training. As important as it is to be conscious of pace in certain runs that are earmarked for pacing skill development, it's equally important to relegate pacing to the back of your mind in other runs. Pacing skill development is meant to be a project, not an obsession. And the overall process should be rewarding, not frustrating, to which end I urge the runners I work with—and you—to focus on the progress that's being made rather than on how far away pacing mastery seems. You can't run free if your running is in any way a burden.

7

Pacing in Competition

There's a reason I define pacing as the art of finding your limit. More than a few great runners over the years have viewed their races as works of art. Steve Prefontaine (yeah, him again) was one such runner, who, while still competing for the University of Oregon, said, "Some people create with words or with music or with a brush and paints. I like to make something beautiful when I run."

It's no accident that the word "performance" is used to refer to what musicians, actors, and other artists do on stage as well as to what runners do in races. For performing artists, there is no amount of rehearsal that guarantees a successful performance before a live audience. It isn't just that they might forget a line or break a string. It's also that, even if everything goes according to script, the performance could be better or worse based on other factors, such as how they're feeling about what they're doing. The greatest performers embrace this uncertainty, relishing the high-stakes nature of performance. They don't want guarantees.

Alas, the same cannot be said of many runners, particularly those who struggle with pacing. Lacking confidence in their ability to solve the unique puzzle that each race presents, these runners would gladly accept an alternate reality in which, if they just did all the necessary work to prepare for a great performance, the performance itself would be automatic. It's a vain wish, however. To find your limit in any given race, you must improvise, working with what you've got that day to feel your way to an outcome that remains undetermined until the moment it happens. Granted, this does mean you have no one but yourself to blame if you blow it. But it also means you get all the credit if you nail it!

Wouldn't you like to create something beautiful when you run? Of course you would. And the only way to do so is to embrace the racing experience as the live solo act that it is. It's like tangoing before a panel of surly judges with a competitive dance partner you've only just met. The many past tangos you've done with other partners will give you a chance to score perfect 10s, but this will only happen if you're able to quickly and effectively read your partner and cooperate with him or her to create a performance that looks rehearsed. Think of each race you do as a new dance partner, and think of those perfect 10s as your personal performance limit on that day.

A good example of what this looks like in the real world comes from Sarah Crouch, an elite runner with whom I did some training during my summer in Flagstaff with NAZ Elite. The following May, Sarah flew to Grand Rapids to race the 2018 USATF 25K Championships. Her last several competitive outings had been disappointing, and four long years had passed since Sarah set a personal best at any distance. Something had to change, and on the eve of the event, Sarah announced that she would compete without a watch, which is not unheard of at the professional level (Galen Rupp left his watch at home when he won the 2020 Olympic Trials Marathon) but was unusual for her. Sarah explained her reasoning as follows in a pre-race interview for FloTrack: "I feel that when I'm wearing a watch I'm constantly looking at it. I'm far too much in my own head. So the goal tomorrow is to race just by instinct, and guts."

Intrigued by the experiment, I tuned in to FloTrack's live coverage the next morning. From the moment Sarah first appeared on my computer screen I knew something special was in the works. She seemed like a different person than the one I had trained with less than a year before, running with a striking combination of aggression and serenity, her eyes focused seemingly miles up the road as she dragged eight-time national champion Aliphine Tuliamuk behind her. Incredibly, Sarah passed the half-marathon mark in 1:12:45, just 35 seconds shy of her four-year-old personal best for that distance, and went on to finish the race in 3rd place. It was a breakthrough performance—Sarah's first podium finish in a national championship race and a huge improvement on her recent racing.

The lesson here is not that runners should never wear watches when they race. In fact, there is no lesson, but through Sarah's story you can see what's possible when a runner fully accepts the performative nature of racing and allows today's limit to guide her to it. Sarah Crouch wasn't just satisfied with her performance in Grand Rapids; she was ecstatically proud of it, and duly so, because she had created it from nothing.

I want you to be ecstatically proud of your future races, and to that end I will devote this chapter to sharing my best advice for pacing in competition. The three most common errors in race pacing are: 1) bad planning (or not having a plan), 2) not sticking to the plan, and 3) sticking too much to the plan. I'll show you how to avoid each of these errors by applying the principles and methods of optimal pacing that you've learned to each unique race experience to create the best possible performance. We will then wrap up by addressing the important difference between racing for time and racing to beat other runners.

BAD PLANNING/NO PLAN

Jim Walmsley came into the 2017 Western States 100-Mile Endurance Run with big ambitions, wanting not just to win the race but to break the course record. The problem was that conditions were not favorable to such an agenda, even for a runner as gifted as Walmsley, who had won the JFK 50 Mile three times and owned the fastest known time (FKT) for crossing the Grand Canyon. A brutal winter had left the early miles of the Western States course in rough shape, with patches of snow still on the ground in many places. Knowing this, the other contenders started out conservatively, marshalling their energy for later in the day, when triple-digit temperatures were expected to add insult to injury. Not Walmsley. Fixated on Timothy Olson's standard of 14:46:44, he covered the first 16 miles just 1 minute slower than he had in his Western States debut the year before, when a heartbreaking wrong turn at 93 miles dropped him from 1st place to an eventual 20th. Already he was nearly 20 minutes ahead of his nearest chaser, and the margin grew steadily from there, stretching to an almost comical 56 minutes at 55 miles, by which point it seemed Walmsley couldn't possibly be caught. And, in fact, he wasn't caught—but that's only because he dropped out at 78 miles, overcooked and exhausted.

Having learned his lesson, Walmsley returned the following year and claimed the course record, then eclipsed his own mark in 2019. And the lesson was this: When you start a race, you need to have a plan—and not just a plan, but a good one. Jim Walmsley's plan to break the Western States 100 course record in 2017 was a bad plan because it failed to factor in the state of the course and the forecasted weather—information that was freely available to everyone and that Walmsley's competitors took full advantage of.

I realize that most runners aren't trying to break course records, but the same planning rules apply to more modest performance goals like beating your own best time in the annual Independence Day 5K road race. The following five rules will help you avoid experiencing the kind of regret Walmsley did.

Consider Pace First, Time Second

The time goals that runners set for races are often somewhat arbitrary. Round numbers in particular exert a pull that causes many to overreach. So, for example, a runner who thinks he's able to run a 5K in about 21 minutes sets a goal to run 20 minutes, and a runner who feels she's in 3:04 marathon shape sets a goal to break 3 hours. I'm oversimplifying a bit to make a point, but you get the idea.

There's nothing wrong with a 21-minute 5K runner dreaming of running a 20-minute 5K, or with a 3:04 marathoner wanting to run a sub-3-hour marathon eventually. The problem is that a runner who's in 21-minute 5K shape today and starts a 5K at a 20-minute pace is likely to finish in 22 minutes, and a runner who's ready to run a 3:04 marathon today and starts out on pace to run 2:59 is likely to finish in 3:14—or not at all. If you want to find your limit in your next race, your goal should be based on a clear-eyed reading of your current ability. This requires that you forget about round numbers, and indeed about finish times in general, for the moment, and instead focus on pace. Ask yourself what is the fastest pace you could sustain for the full distance of your upcoming race, and then use your answer to project a finish time. It's a small difference in orientation but it's far more likely to yield a goal that represents your present limit.

If you're currently the round-number type of goal setter, chances are you haven't put much thought into the process by which you set goals. A certain number just sort of pops into your head a couple of weeks before the race, and it feels about right, so that's your goal. Pace-based goal-setting, by contrast, is infused throughout the entire training process. Day by day, you ask yourself, "What is this run telling me about the fastest pace I could sustain for the full distance of my upcoming race?" As a result, by the time you settle on a final goal, the number you pick has a solid basis. Benchmark workouts are especially helpful in this regard.

Use Benchmark Workouts to Refine Your Goal

As I mentioned in Chapter 6, any run you do can tell you something about your current fitness, but certain workouts tell you more, especially as they relate to an upcoming race. To fulfill their purpose, such benchmark workouts need to have some relevance to the race they precede, and they must also be familiar enough from prior experience to provide a basis for comparisons. Obviously, it helps if the race distance you're targeting is itself at least somewhat familiar as well.

For example, long runs containing extended efforts at anticipated marathon race pace (e.g., 10 miles easy plus 10 miles at marathon pace) are commonly used as a benchmark workout prior to marathon competition. These workouts are challenging enough that they shouldn't be done very often, but even one big marathon-pace workout done before a marathon will give the runner who does it something to go on when interpreting the results of the next big marathon-pace run performed ahead of a second marathon.

Here are examples of useful benchmark workouts for other popular race distances:

5K: 5 × 1K at estimated 5K race pace/400m jog recovery
10K: 6 × 1 mile at estimated 10K race pace/400m jog recovery
Half marathon: 3 × 3 miles (or 5K) at estimated half-marathon pace/1:00 rest

Benchmark workouts don't have to be done at your estimated current pace for a particular race distance. The 5K workout above could serve just as well as a benchmark workout for a 10K race if you've done enough of both. Interval workouts targeting maximal aerobic speed have been used with good success as performance benchmarks for 5K races, as have runs focused on critical velocity by runners training for 10Ks and half marathons. And don't forget about relaxed time trials, as discussed in Chapter 6. The two main criteria for all such runs are relevance and familiarity. Any run becomes familiar with repetition, of course, and relevance is broadly defined in running. Even milers need stamina and even marathoners need speed.

Aim for Incremental Improvements

In 2007, Haile Gebrselassie set a new world record of 2:04:26 in winning the Berlin Marathon. The first thing he said after crossing the finish line was, "I can run faster." The following year, Geb returned to Berlin and bettered his mark, running 2:03:58—precisely 1 second per mile faster than last time.

As this example illustrates, it's easier to know you can go faster than it is to know how fast you can go. In fact, it's infinitely easier, as it is simply impossible for any runner to know how fast he can ultimately go at any race distance. So instead of setting goals based on your best guess as to how fast you can go, just aim for incremental improvement. If, for example, you've run three half marathons and your best and most recent time was 1:44:14, use this number as a baseline for setting your next goal. If your current training suggests you're ready to make a small step forward, then shoot to lower your mark by 1 to 2 seconds per mile. If you've experienced a breakthrough in fitness since your last half, set the bar a little higher.

You don't always have to be fitter to seek incremental improvements. Haile Gebrselassie wasn't any fitter when he set his second marathon world record at age thirty-six than he was when he set his first one the year before. He just had the advantage of having already run a marathon in 2:04:26, which gave him a solid basis for believing he could squeeze a few more seconds out of himself. The beauty of incremental improvement is that, with repetition, it works magic, enabling runners to go faster even after they've stopped getting "better," coaxing them through the last few purely mental steps toward their ultimate limit.

The weakness of the incremental-improvements approach is that it demands patience, and it assumes you'll have many bites at the same apple—whether it's half marathons or anything else. But what if your next race is at a distance you've never done, or you specialize in 100-milers, where you only get so many bites at the apple? In these cases, the incremental-improvements approach won't be as useful. Simple as that.

Consider the Course and Conditions

Jim Walmsley is hardly alone in having failed to properly account for course conditions in setting and pursuing a race time goal. Too many runners set goals that assume an easy course and favorable conditions and then apply that goal to an event that has a less-than-easy course and is likely to take place in less-than-perfect conditions. There's nothing wrong with using a "perfect world" scenario as your starting point in the goal-setting process, but this number should be treated as just that—a starting point—that is subject to future revision based on specific discrepancies (topography, terrain, winds, temperature and humidity, and elevation, in particular) between a perfect world and the one you'll be racing in.

When cyclist Bradley Wiggins broke the world record for the one-hour time trial at a London velodrome in 2015, he adjusted his goal from 16.1 seconds per lap to 16.4 seconds per lap at the last moment based on an unexpectedly high barometric pressure reading. A solo cycling time trial performed in a velodrome is a sufficiently controlled experiment that such precision is possible, whereas in most running events there's a little more guesswork involved. Tools such as the Run S.M.A.R.T. Project's running calculator and Stryd's race prediction feature can help you quantify the anticipated effect of weather and elevation gain on your race pace. Accounting mathematically for other factors, such as strong winds and muddy trails, is more difficult. The runners who do the best job of adjusting their pace to unfavorable conditions of all kinds seldom bother with calculators. Instead they simply start their races with a general expectation of running slower than normal and then *feel* their way to the appropriate pace as they go.

"How is this done?" you ask. It's done the same way good pacing is always done. Runners who succeed in finding their limit despite unfavorable conditions take the race on its own terms, asking themselves throughout it, "Can I sustain this effort the rest of the way?" All runners do this to an extent, but pacing masters do it in a more focused way, actively listening to their perception of effort rather than passively hearing it, as less skilled pacers do. By actively studying their subjective effort, pacing masters not only are better able to answer the all-important sustainability question assuredly but are also able to draw deeper learning from each race, so their answers are even more assured in the next one.

A less skilled pacer cannot instantly become a pacing master by emulating her practice of really tuning in to her effort during races, but she can begin to close the gap in this fashion.

By the way, the correct answer to the question, "Can I sustain this effort the rest of the way?" (as Bradley Wiggins points out in his memoir, *My Hour*), is not "Yes" but "Maybe." Surprised? Think about it: If you answer "Yes" to this question, meaning you're *sure* the effort is sustainable, then you're all but sure to fall short of your real limit. Keep in mind that to succeed in finding your limit in a race is to just barely escape hitting the wall before you finish, and there's just no way to flirt so closely with disaster without running in a state of uncertainty most of the way. The risk of actually hitting the wall with this approach is minimal because the moment the runner's "Maybe" tilts too far in the direction of "No," warning of impending disaster, he slows down immediately, before it's too late. In regulating their effort during races, pacing masters deliberately seek the narrow zone of uncertainty that lies between knowing they can keep up their current pace and knowing they can't. This chosen uncertainty is very different from the cluelessness of the novice runner, who has no earthly idea whether she's running too fast or too slow or just right. It's a definite maybe, if you will. While the runner does not know for sure if she can sustain the effort, she does know that if she's running too fast or too slow, it's not by much.

When a race you're doing is similar in most respects to others of its kind that you've done in the past, you can pace your way through it by regulating your effort based on your knowledge of how you should be feeling at each point along the way. Suppose there's a half marathon you've run twice before, but in your third go at it you're forced to complete it under a heavy downpour. In this case, you'll want to make sure your core effort level is the same at 4 miles, at 7 miles, and so forth as it was in prior dry years (assuming you paced those races well), letting the actual numbers take care of themselves rather than keying off numbers based on some prior calculation.

Such comparative adjustments are less useful in races that are so unique in design that they really can't be compared to other races of the same distance. Kilian Jornet's course record at the Hardrock 100 (22:41:35) is more than 7 hours slower than Jim Walmsley's course record at the Western States 100, not because Jornet is an inferior runner or Hardrock a less competitive race but because the course is far more difficult. A runner who is competing in either of these events for the first time will need to draw upon their experience in a general way when answering the question, "Is this effort sustainable?" When planning for extreme races of this sort, you can set rough expectations for your performance by studying historical results. How have runners of similar ability fared in this particular event in past years? Obtaining this information will make you slightly less reliant on perceptions in the early part of the race.

Don't Be Afraid to Make a Mistake

Having a bad race due to poor pacing is not the end of the world—unless it's the Worlds End Ultramarathon in Pennsylvania's Loyalsock State Forest, in which case it's the end of the world even if your pacing is nearly perfect. Always remember that pacing mistakes are grist for the mill of pacing skill development. Yes, it's disappointing—and sometimes downright painful—to hit the wall in a race as a result of misjudging your limit. But each of these experiences has the potential to teach you a lesson that will help you pace better next time.

I say "has the potential" because learning from pacing errors is not automatic. As the philosopher John Dewey wrote, "We do not learn from experience. . . . We learn from reflecting on experience." To avoid repeating the same pacing mistake over and over, you need to reflect on what you did wrong and then take a conscious intention to do otherwise into your next race. This is where decision tracking comes in. After each race, evaluate your pacing decisions with a critical eye, flag the mistakes, and ask yourself what you could have done differently to produce a better overall performance. You can't go back in time, but you can ensure that history doesn't repeat itself.

NOT STICKING TO THE PLAN

Professional triathlete Jesse Thomas came into the 2016 Ironman World Championship with a solid plan. On the basis of prior experience at the Ironman distance as well as recent training performance, he had identified a power target that he intended to sustain throughout the bike leg. A strong runner (he'd won state championships in track and cross country in high school and earned All-American status in the same sports at Stanford University), Thomas needed to ride hard enough to avoid giving up too much ground to the competition but not so hard that his legs had nothing left for the marathon, and his power target struck this balance.

As I say, it was a sound plan. But when he got out onto the bike course and found himself being left behind by uber-cyclists Sebastian Kienle and Michael Weiss, Thomas cast aside his pre-race strategy and gave chase. Upon reaching the 60-mile mark in the hilltop village of Hawi, Thomas discovered that his average power output up to that point exceeded not just the target he'd set but also his average power in a recent race of half the distance, Ironman 70.3 Santa Cruz.

"And then I just completely crumbled," Thomas told a reporter for *Triathlete* after his disappointing 16th-place finish. "It was a long, long, long day."

Sound familiar? Long days are as common in running as they are in triathlon. All too often, runners arrive at the start line with a well-thought-out pacing plan for the race, only to crumple it up and go faster than intended, whether in reaction to the athletes around them, or as a panic response to an early setback such as having a shoelace come untied, or even just because they feel unexpectedly terrific. Assuming the plan was indeed the right one, such spontaneous departures from script seldom end well, as Jesse Thomas can attest. It's almost as if the you who plans for the race is different from the you who does the race, a less rational version of yourself addled by adrenaline, stress, and competitive juices.

To avoid letting the you who races abandon the plan created by the you who prepares, take a cue from brave Ulysses, that hero of ancient Greek literature. In Homer's *Odyssey*, Ulysses resists falling prey to the Sirens' song by having himself tied to the mast of his boat. That is essentially what you need to do to yourself in committing to your pacing plan for the next race. Take a mental step back from the plan itself and vow to stick to it unless something happens during the race that truly requires you to make an adjustment. This note to your future self will bind you to the mast of your plan when you're tempted to stray from it.

An historical counterpoint to Jesse Thomas's long, long, long day at the 2016 Ironman World Championship was Mark Allen's performance at the same event nineteen years earlier. It was Allen's swan song as a professional triathlete, a do-or-die attempt to match his former rival Dave Scott's record of six world titles at age thirty-seven. Allen's plan for the bike leg was to keep his heart rate at or below 150 beats per minute, a number that, like Thomas's power target, he'd arrived at through experience. In the early miles, Allen lost his lead to a pair of younger Germans, the strongest of whom, Thomas "Hell on Wheels" Hellriegel, eventually built a seemingly insurmountable advantage of 13:31 over the five-time champion. But the reason Allen fell so far behind wasn't that he couldn't go faster. Rather, he lost ground because he chose not to go faster, knowing that sticking to his plan gave him the best chance of winning, regardless of what anyone else did. Resisting the temptation to push harder wasn't easy, but Allen's Ulysses-like discipline was rewarded when a grimacing Hellriegel cracked during the marathon and Allen slid past him and into history.

Remember Mark Allen the next time you're tempted to crumple up your pacing plan mid-race.

STICKING TOO MUCH TO THE PLAN

I'll stop picking on Jesse Thomas in a minute, but before I do I'd like to share something that was said by the winner of the 2016 Ironman World Championship, Jan Frodeno, who finished more than 26 minutes ahead of Thomas on that long, long, long day. "On race day," Frodeno told Slowtwitch reporter Timothy Carlson, "statistics and numbers all really go to shit." In other words, you can plan all you want, but you'd better be ready to improvise if the reality you confront in the race is different from the one your plan assumed.

At first blush, Frodeno's sentiment might seem to contradict the advice I just gave you to stick to your pacing plan in races, as Mark Allen did so successfully in 1997. But remember the qualifier: "unless something happens during the race that truly requires you to make an adjustment." It was this caveat that Frodeno was referring to in his colorful post-race remark. To find your limit in a race, you must first have a good plan, and then you must have the discipline to resist emotionally driven temptations to abandon the plan, but you must also be willing to depart from your target numbers if circumstances create a need to do so. And, as Jan Frodeno would tell you, in most races it becomes necessary at some point to improvise, at least in small ways.

I'll give you a personal example of the consequences of sticking to a plan too stubbornly and the rewards of improvising intelligently mid-race. In 2002, I ran the Long Beach Marathon in the hope of finishing in 2:45, or 1 minute faster than my personal best. I started at the required pace of 6:18 per mile and held it consistently as I made my way through the pancake-flat course, but around mile 8 the pace began to feel harder than it should have, and my gut told me to slow down. But a second instinct overruled my gut and I stuck to the plan, with the result that I hit the wall at 21 miles and walked the last 3 miles, finishing in 3:11:16.

Seven years later, I ran the Silicon Valley Marathon with the goal of finishing in 2:39, having recently recorded a half-marathon time that made this goal very reasonable. I started the race at the required pace of 6:05 per mile and held it consistently, but around mile 6 the pace began to feel harder than it should have, and my gut told me to slow down. Right on cue, a second instinct urged me to press on. This time, however, I heeded my gut and eased back to a pace that felt more realistic. The result was that, at 21 miles, I had enough energy left to speed up again, and I finished in 2:41:29, missing my goal but still achieving a new personal best.

Remember that the purpose of a pacing plan is not to carry it out no matter what but to help you achieve a successful race, and be open to the possibility that achieving a successful race will require you to modify or even abandon your plan on the fly. These decisions aren't always easy. Sometimes it's hard to know which voice to trust among those squabbling inside your head. I doubt I would have made the good decision I did in the Silicon Valley Marathon if I hadn't made bad decisions like the one I made in the Long Beach Marathon seven years earlier. Your chances of making the right decision in these difficult moments will be greater if you understand exactly what's happening in them, as you now do.

RACING FOR POSITION

If you want a better understanding of the difference between racing for time, which has been our topic up to this point, and racing for position, which entails trying to finish ahead of other runners, watch the 2016 Olympics men's 1500m final. The metric mile, as it is known, goes all the way back to the first modern Olympics in 1896, and is almost always a tactical affair, which is a diplomatic way of saying slow. That's because the person who is leading after the first or second of the race's 3.75 total laps seldom wins, so nobody wants to lead and the pace suffers accordingly. But this particular race was an extreme case.

American Matthew Centrowitz came to Rio as the reigning indoor world champion and a strong medal contender. As such, he did not want to bear the burden of leading any more than the other finalists, but that's precisely where he found himself after the usual sprint for position over the first 100 meters. Centro's medal aspirations were far from dashed at this point, but they soon would be if he either ran too hard and used up all his energy while allowing the other runners to cruise in his slipstream or ran too slow and allowed himself to get boxed in by competitors passing him on the outside. The solution he arrived at was to run slow enough (66 seconds for lap one, 69 seconds for lap two) to tempt other racers to pass him and then abruptly speed up each time a runner tried to do so.

The result was one of the most tactically brilliant running performances I have ever witnessed. Knowing that his competitors were only willing to gamble so much on a bid to seize the lead before the last lap, Centro accelerated as much as necessary to cause each succeeding aspirant to think better of it and fall back. His own gamble was to exert the least effort possible to retain the lead no matter what, even going so far as to throw a couple of elbows at indoor 1000m world record holder Ayanleh Souleiman as he tried to overtake the American in lap three.

Predictably, all hell broke loose when the bell rang, signaling the final lap. Now everyone was willing to risk everything to pass Centrowitz, who was no less motivated to fight them off, and though Souleiman was able to briefly nose ahead of him on the outside, he couldn't close the deal by moving to the rail, and within seconds Centro was back ahead, where he remained all the way to the finish. His winning formula was utterly original—leading from the very first step until he stopped the clock at 3:50.00, a time that would be surpassed three weeks later by the top four finishers in the final of the Paralympic men's 1500m T13.

The three keys to racing successfully for position—all exemplified by Matthew Centrowitz's Rio performance—are: 1) playing to your strengths, 2) using the runners you're trying to beat to your own best advantage, and 3) running *your* race.

Play to Your Strengths

Playing to your strengths is important because each runner has a different combination of strengths and weaknesses than other runners of similar overall ability. Hence, if you want to finish ahead of them in a race, you must try to neutralize their strengths with yours. I used to coach a trail runner who had a preternatural gift for bombing down technical descents at high speeds without face-planting. Recognizing this strength, we strategized in a way that enabled him to win races by dropping competitors on early descents and using later descents to overtake competitors he'd allowed to get away from him on preceding climbs and flatter sections. Consider your relative strengths as a runner and how to exploit them in individual races against particular competitors you'll face at those events.

Use Other Runners

In everyday life, it is considered unscrupulous to use other people. In competitive running, however, you're a sucker if you don't! Think of the runners you're trying to beat as objects that you can manipulate in certain ways to increase your chances of finishing ahead of them. An extreme example of this mentality comes from my friend and fellow running coach James McKirdy, who was one of Connecticut's top decathletes in his high school days. In his senior outdoor track season, McKirdy came into the final event of the state championship—the 1500-meter run—in 3rd place, 113 points behind leader Josh Fournier and needing to beat him soundly to claim the title. Prior to the race, McKirdy's coach told him to forget everything he knew about smart pacing and run the first lap ridiculously fast, knowing that Fournier, who was more of a sprint specialist, would mark him closely and pay the price later. More than willing to give this unconventional strategy a try, McKirdy completed the opening 400-meter circuit in 61 seconds (or 5 seconds faster than Matthew Centrowitz in the 2016 Olympics), with Fournier glued to his heels. Sure enough, as McKirdy lost steam, Fournier imploded, eventually staggering across the finish line 33 seconds behind the wily winner.

As a coach today, James McKirdy defines "racing" (meaning racing for position) as affecting how someone else performs with your decisions. This is exactly what I mean by using other runners to your own best advantage. The example I just provided is over-the-top, but there are lots of other specific decision types that you can use to affect the performance of other runners in competition. These include surging to test the legs of a competitor you're currently matching strides with, tucking in behind other runners to let them do the extra work of blocking the wind and setting the pace, masking your discomfort behind a poker face to sow doubt in the mind of a competitor, and exaggerating your discomfort (i.e., playing possum) to make another runner overconfident before you strike.

Run Your Race

The flip side of controlling other runners in such ways is not allowing them to control you. Running your own race means pacing your race in a way that best serves your competitive interests regardless of what your competitors do. I witnessed a good example of this strategy at the 2007 USATF Cross Country Championships in Boulder, Colorado. Dathan Ritzenhein took the men's senior race out hard, breaking away from the lead pack just 1 km into the 12K race. Alan Culpepper, judging the pace too aggressive, elected to let him go, a decision that resulted in Ritzenhein gapping him by 20 seconds over the next 3 km. But in lap four of six, Ritz began to falter, and Culpepper's self-control was rewarded with a dominating 26-second victory.

In the heat of battle, it can be difficult to make the correct split-second decision in reaction (or nonreaction) to something another runner does. In some instances, it's in your best interest to cover a competitor's surge; in others, it's best to let the runner go. You won't always make the right decision, but if you run each race with the intent to control your performance regardless of others' actions, and if you use post-race decision tracking to assess your tactical decisions, you will eventually get to a place where you almost always do the right thing.

8

Macro Pacing

In February 2020 I flew to Atlanta to watch the U.S. Olympic Team Trials Women's and Men's Marathons. I wasn't the only fan of elite American running who made the pilgrimage. Tens of thousands of my fellow devotees crowded the sidewalks to witness big names like Galen Rupp and Des Linden as well as up-and-comers including Jake Riley and Molly Seidel take their best shot at qualifying for the Tokyo Olympics. It was a thrilling experience, and among the biggest thrills for me, as a forty-eight-year-old, still-competitive runner, was seeing forty-three-year-old Abdi Abdirahman qualify for his fifth Olympics with a 3rd-place finish in the men's race.

I had followed Abdi's career from the beginning, and I had even run with him a few years earlier, so I wasn't quite as surprised as some people were by his performance in Atlanta. I knew the answer to the question many folks were asking about Abdi after the race: "What's his secret?"

In a word: pacing.

Until this point I've been writing as if pacing happens only within individual runs, but that's only one kind of pacing, which we can now classify as *micro pacing*. If micro pacing is the "goal-directed distribution and management of effort across the duration of an exercise bout," *macro pacing* is the goal-directed distribution of effort across a full training cycle, an entire competitive running career, or even a lifetime. Within a single run, pacing enables a runner to find his present limit. Over longer time spans, a slightly different application of the same basic aptitude allows runners like Abdi Abdirahman to reach and sustain their *ultimate* limit.

Macro pacing is not simply an extended version of race pacing, however. Side-by-side graphs of optimal race pacing and optimal career pacing would look rather different. In race pacing, as we know, the watchword is steadiness. A graph of a well-paced race takes the shape of a horizontal line with gentle undulations and perhaps a spike at the very end marking the finishing kick. A graph of Abdi Abdirahman's entire running career, by contrast, would look more like an upward sloping sine wave, with sharp dips indicating the three- to four-week breaks he took after each training cycle, occasional peaks representing periods when he was doing as much work as his body could absorb (like when I met him a few weeks before the 2017 New York City Marathon), and longer, flattish segments between these peaks and valleys representing an overall pattern of consistency (week after week, month after month, and year after year of speed sessions every Tuesday or Wednesday, tempo runs every Friday, and long runs every Sunday). In short, effective macro pacing is a matter of being steady *but not too steady.* If condensed into a single run, the career of Abdirahman and every other runner who just keeps rolling along, season after season, would take the form of a brisk jog broken up by brief accelerations to full speed and occasional dead stops.

You don't have to be Abdi Abdirahman to make five Olympic teams. Wait a minute—yes, you do! That's not what I meant to say. What I meant to say is that most of the macro pacing errors runners make can be avoided by following the example of runners like Abdi. If you were to receive advice on macro pacing directly from such a runner, they would tell you five things:

1. Be patient.
2. Don't get greedy.
3. Be balanced.
4. Don't let yourself go.
5. Stay in love.

My advice is the same, though I might need more words to express it.

BE PATIENT

Sara Hall ran her first marathon in Los Angeles in 2015, one month before her 33rd birthday. Hall was then well along in a successful professional running career that included appearances at the Pan Am Games, the World Indoor Championships, and the World Cross Country Championships. But the marathon is a different animal. Struck by leg cramps in the middle miles, she hobbled across the finish line in 2:48:02.

Eight months later, in Chicago, Hall improved her marathon time to 2:31:14. The following year, she took another minute off her personal best. In 2017, she lowered her PB twice more, going from 2:28:26 in Tokyo to 2:27:21 in Frankfurt. Hall's lone marathon in 2018, held in out-of-the-way Ottawa, was yet another incremental improvement: 2:26:19. In Berlin the next fall she dropped her time to 2:22:16, and in 2020, at age 37, Hall won The Marathon Project in 2:20:32, the second-fastest time ever run by an American woman.

After setting the last of these marks, Hall told *New York Times* writer Lindsay Crouse, "We can be an instant-gratification culture, but I've had to cultivate a long-term approach to my career. I figured as long as I could keep working on my craft, chipping away, finding joy in the mundane, then that had to be enough." This patient mindset is a requirement for successful macro pacing. Progress can't be rushed in running. Improvement often does come quickly in the beginning, but years of methodical "chipping away" (a phrase that was also used by macro pacing master Ben Bruce in reference to his own progression) are required to fulfill the last few percent of a runner's potential.

Running tends to attract patient people and to cultivate patience in the people it attracts. It's not patience most runners lack but rather an understanding of how to exercise their patience to achieve long-term improvement. Sara Hall lowered her marathon time by 28 minutes over a span of five years. Stated like that, it seems like a big leap, but Hall didn't make any leaps in the process of fulfilling her marathon potential. She did not attempt to radically increase her training load or rethink her whole approach to training in search of enormous improvements. Instead, she learned from each marathon cycle, applied what she learned to the next one, and raised the bar a little higher. This is the right formula for manifesting patience in the career arc of any runner.

DON'T GET GREEDY

Drew Hunter returned home to Boulder, Colorado, from Oslo, Norway, in June 2019 with a shiny new PB of 7:39 for 3000 meters and plenty of time to rest a sore right foot he'd acquired while in Europe before he sharpened up for the USATF Outdoor Championships in late July. But the twenty-one-year-old was so hyped up about his soaring fitness that instead of resting he dove straight back into heavy training, with predictable results. Within a few weeks Hunter's foot pain had intensified to the point where he was forced to reduce his run frequency to three times per week. Remarkably, he was still able to qualify for the World Championships in the 5000-meter event, but when he went out to celebrate the achievement with his teammates, he couldn't even put weight on the foot, and he was later forced to withdraw from worlds.

"The biggest thing I've learned this year is to not get too greedy with mileage," Hunter told *Runner's World* writer Hailey Middlebrook in the wake of this disappointment. "Runners have this mindset that more is always better, and that if I'm doing well on 'X' mileage, that I'll be even faster if I do more. But that's not the case."

The British phrase "purple patch" refers to a period when everything is going right for an athlete. They're nailing every workout, feeling fit, and enjoying the process. It is extremely tempting at these times to keep pushing for more, but doing so almost always leads to regret. Purple patches never last long. They can't, because they occur when a runner is very close to peak fitness, which is not a sustainable state. Too often, runners become intoxicated by how well they are running and make a bad decision, either training harder to see if they can get even fitter or ignoring signs that their body is at its limit (as Drew Hunter did).

When a purple patch is well timed, a runner is able to complete her peak race in good health and with supreme fitness. But some then get greedy, and try to extend their purple patch, teeing up another race to run when they should follow Abdi Abdirahman's example and take a break. These efforts to milk a fitness peak rarely turn out well.

It is only human to get excited when you're killing it in training. But a part of you should also be wary when you enter a purple patch. Know that it can't last long. Enjoy the experience and don't risk spoiling it, or worse, delaying your next opportunity to hit a purple patch, by trying to go for more.

BE BALANCED

There is a common misconception that the greatest athletes are completely obsessed with their sport and make little room in their lives for anything else. Although some such athletes do exist, most of the top runners I've gotten to know are strikingly balanced. A good example is Kellyn Taylor, another member of the NAZ Elite team with whom I trained in 2017. Taylor is also a good example of a macro-pacing master, having set her personal-best times for 5000 meters, 10,000 meters, the half marathon, and the marathon between the ages of 31 and 34 after achieving no small measure of success earlier in her career.

The furthest thing from a running geek, Kellyn puts the sport completely out of mind when she's not actively engaged in it. Her top priority is parenting her daughter, Kylyn, who was born when Kellyn was just getting started in her professional running career, as well as a number of foster children she and her husband, Kyle, have taken into their home over the years. During the time I spent with Taylor and her teammates in Flagstaff, she was deeply immersed in training to become a professional firefighter, a commitment that absorbed tremendous amounts of time and energy. Understandably, Taylor was usually the last runner to arrive for a team workout and the first one to leave after completing it.

You might think this busy, multidimensional lifestyle would be a recipe for poor running, but Taylor's results speak for themselves. And although I can't think of another elite runner who is also a firefighter and a foster parent, balanced human beings are the norm at the highest level of all sports, not just running. Evidence of this comes from an analysis conducted by the Australian Institute of Sport's Personal Excellence program, which focuses on the holistic development of athletes with the goal of maximizing their overall well-being. Program director Megan Fritsch gathered information on the makeup and performance of the Australian Olympic Team in the 2008 and 2012 Summer Games. Interestingly, she found that in both Beijing and London student-athletes were more likely than other athletes to win medals, with student athletes accounting for 40 percent of the 2012 Australian Olympic team and 63 percent of the medals brought home from London. Of course, student-athlete status is not a guarantee of life-sport balance, but it is a serviceable stand-in for the purposes of this type of analysis.

The idea that caring a little less about running and a little more about other parts of life yields better long-term running performance is somewhat counterintuitive. How does it work? Psychologists who've looked at this question have identified a few different answers. One is simply that balanced athletes are happier, and happier people perform better in any activity they're passionate about. Athletes are human beings, after all, not exercise machines, and human beings have many facets. An athlete can pretend he has only one facet by focusing exclusively on one of them—sport—but the fact of the matter is that he does have other facets, which then whither from neglect, weakening the foundation of overall well-being that athletic performance depends on.

In an interview conducted after he won the 1974 Commonwealth Games Marathon, English runner Ian Thompson said, "I was happy about a lot of other things in life besides my running. Everything was clicking, and I was in a relaxed frame of mind—which is ideal." These words hold true for every runner. If you want to run your very best, you must fit running into your life in a way that makes you happy with a lot of other things besides your running. In fact, the mere temptation to allow running to completely dominate a person's life is a pretty good indication that the person isn't happy in the first place. Submitting to this temptation will only make things worse. I've been known to tell my athletes that if all they care about is running, their best move is to start caring about other things, because doing so will aid their running.

Becoming unbalanced in the direction of sport also tends to negatively impact self-esteem and confidence, which in turn harms performance. A bad race is less likely to strike a blow to a runner's self-esteem and confidence if that race comes the day after the runner aced a chemistry exam or was named Employee of the Week or saw her son give his first piano recital. As these examples show, runners with balanced lives have more sources of positive self-esteem and confidence than runners whose identity is completely enmeshed in the sport. In much the same way that a diverse stock portfolio reduces the risk of being dragged down financially by one bad investment, having a balanced life reduces the risk of being dragged down emotionally by disappointment or failure in one area.

Balanced runners are also at a lower risk of overdoing their training. It's easy to see why. Suppose you quit your job for the sake of turning pro and focusing exclusively on running. The first week is likely to be dominated by feelings of excitement, freedom, and hope. But by Thursday of week two you might find yourself sitting on the sofa at three o'clock in the afternoon, bored, having already run twice, lifted weights, and stretched, and think, *I suppose it couldn't hurt to kill some time with a little light cross-training....*

This is why actual professional runners like Kellyn Taylor maintain balanced lives despite having the freedom to go all-in with running. Taylor doesn't have time to overtrain. Heck, she doesn't even have time (or at least doesn't feel she has time) for the fancy mobility exercises that her teammates and other elite runners do before every run. She just shows up and goes, which might not be the best thing from a purely physiological perspective, but again, her results speak for themselves.

Beyond making it harder to overtrain, having a rich life outside of running increases training efficiency. When you have only so much time and energy to devote to your training, you are motivated to make the most of every minute. It's a version of Parkinson's Law—the idea that one's work expands to fill the time available to get it done. Aware that the obverse is true too, savvy corporations use project deadlines and time restrictions as a means to force employees to tighten up their practices in ways that increase the overall quality of their work. You can do the same with your training by strictly compartmentalizing running in the context of your life. As the saying goes, "If you want to get something done, ask a busy person."

DON'T LET YOURSELF GO

In the winter of 1987, when I was a junior in high school, I competed in an indoor track meet at Dartmouth College. Word got out during the meet that the legendary Henry Rono would be taking part in an open 5000-meter race after the kids were finished competing. Already a huge fan of the sport, I knew all about Rono, who in 1978 had broken four world records at distances ranging from 3000 meters to 10,000 meters in the span of eighty-one days. Alcoholism soon derailed his career, but at age thirty-four Rono had committed himself to staging a comeback, and the indoor 5000-meter race that I forced my entire team to hang around and watch instead of getting started on the long bus ride back home was his first rust buster.

It did not go well. Rono started out okay, pushing the pace up front with Jersey boy Marty Ludwikowski, but he never looked comfortable, and within a few laps he'd begun to fall back. Having clocked 13:06 for the same distance nine years earlier, he finished 8th in 14:38. His comeback fizzled not long thereafter.

Henry Rono's story is a cautionary tale for runners who want to run well not just today but also tomorrow, and ten years from now. It goes without saying that if you try to push hard all the time, you're not likely to perform at or near peak level for years on end. But longevity in the sport is just as unlikely if you back off too much, to the point of "letting yourself go," or dig yourself into a hole that's hard to get out of. Rono's alcoholism is an extreme example of the phenomenon, but there are less extreme and more common ways of letting one-self go that are also harmful to macro pacing.

Take my brother Josh. Three years older than me, Josh started running at the same time I did, a few years before my close encounter with Henry Rono. We were closely matched in ability, our PBs only a few seconds apart at a variety of distances. But whereas I kept running throughout my 20s, 30s, and 40s, Josh went for long stretches without ever lacing up his shoes and gained a lot of weight during these periods. Consequently, when at age forty-eight he embarked on a quest to qualify for the Boston Marathon, it took him seemingly forever to excavate his talent from underneath the layers of disuse it was buried under. He got there eventually, but he often regretted those years of letting himself go.

I want to emphasize that the message here is not that you should never place running on life's back burner. Just be sure not to remove it from the stovetop entirely if you have any intention of racing well in the future.

STAY IN LOVE

Although I saved this fifth "rule" of macro pacing for last, I think it's the most important one. If you spend time talking to a dozen runners who have succeeded in performing at or near their ultimate limit for a long time, the most striking shared quality you will see in them is a great passion for running. For proof, look no further than our friend Abdi Abdirahman, who told *PodiumRunner's* Hannah Borenstein before the 2020 Olympic Trials, "I love running. It's my hobby."

When an experienced runner continues to enjoy running year after year as much as he did when he first fell in love with the sport, he invariably finds ways to keep running well. All too often, though, that initial thrill dissipates over time, and running becomes a mere habit maintained by its own inertia rather than by the force of passion. It's no tragedy for a runner to fall out of love with running and trade it for golf or rock climbing, but it is sad when a runner keeps putting the same amount of energy into her running as she did during the courting phase but no longer feels she's getting the same return in enjoyment.

When the thrill does fade, it does so for one of two reasons: loss of balance or an excessive focus on outcomes (i.e., goals) at the expense of the process of pursuing goals. Oftentimes the two phenomena go hand in hand, with an excessive focus on outcomes leading to an unhealthy run/life balance. We've discussed the importance of balance already, so let's now talk about the importance of maintaining a process focus as a runner.

In 2020 I was contacted via Instagram by Cat Bradley, a professional ultrarunner who was looking for a new coach to help her with her mental game. Three years earlier, Cat had been the surprise winner of the Western States 100-Mile Endurance Run as a twenty-five-year-old full-time kindergarten teacher. The victory changed Cat's life, landing her a shoe sponsor and enabling her to quit her job and focus on running. But with these changes came new expectations, a perceived pressure to follow up her Western States performance with similar achievements. Almost before she knew it, Cat had allowed her focus to slip from racing for the thrill of competition to racing only to win, and her performance suffered as a result. At the time she reached out to me, Cat had just come off a nine-week break from running, during which she contemplated quitting the sport.

During our first phone conversation, I asked Cat what she feared most.

"I'm afraid I'll never love racing again," she answered, choking up.

In response to this, I suggested we make it her number-one goal for the upcoming competitive season to have as much fun as possible.

"Pretend there's a huge cash prize that will be handed out at the end of the year to the runner who has the most fun," I said, "and go after it with a laser focus."

In proposing this mindset, I was not suggesting to Cat that she give up on trying to win races. She was a professional runner, after all, and as such she was literally paid to win races. Rather, I wanted her to focus on having fun because I believed that doing so would give her the best chance of returning to the competitive mountaintop. Science supports this belief. Sports psychology research has repeatedly shown that athletes tend to perform better when they focus more on the process of chasing desired outcomes than on the outcomes themselves, and that enjoying the process is inextricably linked to maintaining a process focus. I think this is what Abdi Abdirahman was getting at when he referred to running as his hobby. Approaching the sport as more of a pastime than a job actually enabled him to do the job better.

Maintaining a process focus is itself a process. There are lots of little tricks you can use to reel your mind back to the present moment when it tries to cast itself ahead to the desired endpoint, usually with a degree of anxiety. Before her first race of 2021, I asked Cat—who keeps a daily journal—to reflect on and write about what it meant to her to compete as the best version of herself. Whatever she came up with would be her goal for the race, to the exclusion of any and all outcome goals. On race day, Cat's rustiness showed, and she ended up in 3rd place, but she succeeded in competing as the best version of herself and came away from the experience feeling happy—far happier than she would have been with the same result one year earlier. And the next time she competed, using the same mindset, Cat won.

This is just one example of the type of method you can use to run better by working on staying in love with running, but there are many others, including self-reminder mantras such as the oldie but goodie, "Run the mile you're in." The main thing is to get in the habit of catching yourself in those moments when your mind tries to leap ahead to the endpoint so you can deploy whichever particular method is most appropriate for the situation.

To the extent that you succeed in shifting your focus from outcomes to the process, you will feel liberated, as though an invisible burden has been lifted from your shoulders. When you're focused on outcomes, you're essentially saying, "I will be happy if and only if I achieve my goal," a mindset that causes the quality of your running experience to depend on something over which you have only partial control. But when you're focused on the process, you're saying to yourself, "I'm going to enjoy doing my best in this run, win or lose," a mindset that puts you in total control of the quality of your experience.

Recently I attended a running camp where I met a runner named Traci who had recently suffered through a disastrous first ultramarathon and was having trouble moving past it.

"What's the point?" she asked me rhetorically. "You train for months to achieve a goal, and then you fall flat on your face and it all seems wasted."

"It sounds like you want a guarantee of success every time you start a race," I said. "But do you really? How much would success really mean if you couldn't fail?"

"I guess you're right," Traci conceded.

Lots of runners think they want guaranteed success, but there's very little satisfaction to be gleaned from a successful outcome when the true credit belongs not to the runner herself but to some outside guarantee . . . or a sports watch. What runners like Traci really want is not guaranteed success but to be in control of their performance—to not need an omnipotent smartwatch or any other form of outside help to run a race they're proud of.

At the beginning of this book I claimed that the most satisfying experience you can have as a competitive runner is knowing what you can do and then going out and doing it. The feeling of self-determination that comes with this knowledge makes the entire race experience enjoyable, regardless of outcome, and it is available only to those who master the skill of pacing, at both levels, micro and macro—for this and only this can free a runner from all external dependencies. Aristotle wrote that true happiness belongs to the self-sufficient, and he was right. The true winner among competitive runners is not the swiftest but the happiest, and the happiest runner is the freest runner, and the freest runner is the runner who has most fully mastered the art of finding his or her limit.

9

5K Training Plans

The four training plans presented in this chapter are designed to help runners master the art of pacing and find their limit at the 5K distance. The various levels cover the needs of everyone from first-timers to elites. Refer back to Chapter 6 for details on the RPE-based intensity scale used throughout the plans and for full explanations of certain terms and workout types. Online versions of the plans are available for separate purchase on the 80/20 Endurance website. Additionally, device-compatible free versions of the individual workouts can be found at 8020endurance.com/on-pace-workouts.

5K

This plan is appropriate for beginning runners preparing for their first 5K event and for more experienced runners who need or prefer a relatively low-volume training program for any reason. Before starting the plan, be sure to build your training to the point where you're comfortably able to run five days a week for up to 30 minutes.

	MONDAY	TUESDAY	WEDNESDAY	THURSDAY
1	Rest	**Fartleks** 5:00 at RPE 2–3 5:00 at RPE 3–4 6 × 0:20 at RPE 8–9 / 1:40 at RPE 2–3 10:00 at RPE 3–4	**Foundation Run** 5:00 at RPE 2–3 15:00 at RPE 3–4	Rest
2	Rest	**Fartleks** 5:00 at RPE 2–3 5:00 at RPE 3–4 4 × 1:00 at RPE 7–8 / 2:00 at RPE 2–3 10:00 at RPE 3–4	**Foundation Run** 5:00 at RPE 2–3 20:00 at RPE 3–4	Rest
3	Rest	**Hill Repetitions** 5:00 at RPE 2–3 5:00 at RPE 3–4 6 × 0:30* uphill at RPE 8–9 / 1:30 at RPE 2–3 10:00 at RPE 2–3 *Stretch Intervals*	**Foundation Run** 5:00 at RPE 2–3 20:00 at RPE 3–4	Rest
4	Rest	**VO₂max Intervals** 5:00 at RPE 2–3 5:00 at RPE 3–4 4 × 2:00* at RPE 7–8 / 1:00 at RPE 2–3 10:00 at RPE 2–3 *Precision Splitting*	**Foundation Run** 5:00 at RPE 2–3 25:00 at RPE 3–4	Rest
5	Rest	**Speed Intervals** 5:00 at RPE 2–3 5:00 at RPE 3–4 6 × 1:00* at RPE 8–9 / 2:00 at RPE 2–3 10:00 at RPE 2–3 *Stretch Intervals*	**Foundation Run** 5:00 at RPE 2–3 25:00 at RPE 3–4	Rest

LEVEL

SSP Steady State Pace
LTP Lactate Threshold Pace
CV Critical Velocity
MAS Maximal Aerobic Speed

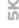

5K

FRIDAY	SATURDAY	SUNDAY
Progression Run 5:00 at RPE 2–3 10:00 at RPE 3–4 8:00 at SSP 4:00 at LTP 2:00 at CV 5:00 at RPE 2–3	**Foundation Run** 5:00 at RPE 2–3 15:00 at RPE 3–4	**Endurance Run** 5:00 at RPE 2–3 20:00 at RPE 3–4 5:00 at RPE 5–6
Progression Run 5:00 at RPE 2–3 20:00 at RPE 3–4 4:00 at LTP 2:00 at CV 1:00 at MAS 5:00 at RPE 2–3	**Foundation Run** 5:00 at RPE 2–3 20:00 at RPE 3–4	**Endurance Run** 5:00 at RPE 2–3 25:00 at RPE 3–4 5:00 at RPE 5–6
Fartleks 5:00 at RPE 2–3 5:00 at RPE 3–4 1:00 at CV, 1:00 at RPE 2–3 2:00 at LTP, 1:00 at RPE 2–3 3:00 at SSP, 1:00 at RPE 2–3 2:00 at LTP, 1:00 at RPE 2–3 1:00 at CV, 1:00 at RPE 2–3 10:00 at RPE 3–4	**Foundation Run** 5:00 at RPE 2–3 20:00 at RPE 3–4	**Endurance Run** 5:00 at RPE 2–3 20:00 at RPE 3–4 5:00 at RPE 5–6
Tempo Run 5:00 at RPE 2–3 5:00 at RPE 3–4 10:00 at RPE 6 5:00 at RPE 2–3 10:00 at RPE 6 10:00 at RPE 2–3	**Foundation Run** 5:00 at RPE 2–3 25:00 at RPE 3–4	**Endurance Run** 5:00 at RPE 2–3 30:00 at RPE 3–4 5:00 at RPE 5–6
Critical Velocity Intervals 5:00 at RPE 2–3 5:00 at RPE 3–4 4 × 4:00* at RPE 6–7 / 2:00 at RPE 2–3 10:00 at RPE 2–3 *Precision Splitting*	**Foundation Run** 5:00 at RPE 2–3 25:00 at RPE 3–4	**Endurance Run** 5:00 at RPE 2–3 35:00 at RPE 3–4 5:00 at RPE 5–6

	MONDAY	TUESDAY	WEDNESDAY	THURSDAY
6	Rest	**Accelerations** 5:00 at RPE 2–3 5:00 at RPE 3–4 11:00 acceleration 10:00 at RPE 2–3 3:00 acceleration 10:00 at RPE 2–3	**Foundation Run** 5:00 at RPE 2–3 25:00 at RPE 3–4	Rest
7	Rest	**VO₂max Intervals** 5:00 at RPE 2–3 5:00 at RPE 3–4 5 × 2:00* at RPE 7–8 / 1:00 at RPE 2–3 10:00 at RPE 2–3 *Precision Splitting*	**Foundation Run** 5:00 at RPE 2–3 30:00 at RPE 3–4	Rest
8	Rest	**Relaxed Time Trial** 1 km at RPE 2–3 1 km at RPE 3–4 5 km at 95% effort 1:00 rest 2 km at RPE 2–3	**Foundation Run** 5:00 at RPE 2–3 30:00 at RPE 3–4	Rest
9	Rest	**Fartleks** 5:00 at RPE 2–3 5:00 at RPE 3–4 6 × 1:00 at RPE 7–8 / 2:00 at RPE 2–3 10:00 at RPE 3–4	Rest	**Fast Finish Run** 5:00 at RPE 2–3 15:00 at RPE 3–4 5:00 at CV

FRIDAY	SATURDAY	SUNDAY
Progression Run	**Foundation Run**	**Endurance Run**
5:00 at RPE 2–3	5:00 at RPE 2–3	5:00 at RPE 2–3
25:00 at RPE 3–4	25:00 at RPE 3–4	25:00 at RPE 3–4
4:00 at LTP		5:00 at RPE 5–6
2:00 at CV		
1:00 at MAS		
5:00 at RPE 2–3		
Tempo Run	**Foundation Run**	**Endurance Run**
5:00 at RPE 2–3	5:00 at RPE 2–3	5:00 at RPE 2–3
5:00 at RPE 3–4	30:00 at RPE 3–4	40:00 at RPE 3–4
12:00 at RPE 6		5:00 at RPE 5–6
5:00 at RPE 2–3		
12:00 at RPE 6		
10:00 at RPE 2–3		
Critical Velocity Intervals	**Foundation Run**	**Endurance Run**
5:00 at RPE 2–3	5:00 at RPE 2–3	5:00 at RPE 2–3
5:00 at RPE 3–4	30:00 at RPE 3–4	45:00 at RPE 3–4
5 × 4:00* at RPE 6–7 / 2:00 at RPE 2–3		5:00 at RPE 5–6
10:00 at RPE 2–3		
Precision Splitting		
Foundation Run	**5K Race**	Rest
5:00 at RPE 2–3		
15:00 at RPE 3–4		

5K

This plan was designed for runners who are ready to take their training load up a notch in order to improve their 5K time. Before starting the plan, be sure to build your training to the point where you're comfortably able to run six days a week for up to 40 minutes.

	MONDAY	TUESDAY	WEDNESDAY	THURSDAY
1	Rest	**Fartleks** 5:00 at RPE 2–3 5:00 at RPE 3–4 6 × 0:20 at RPE 8–9 / 1:40 at RPE 2–3 10:00 at RPE 3–4	**Foundation Run** 5:00 at RPE 2–3 25:00 at RPE 3–4	**Foundation Run** 5:00 at RPE 2–3 25:00 at RPE 3–4
2	Rest	**Fartleks** 5:00 at RPE 2–3 5:00 at RPE 3–4 6 × 1:00 at RPE 7–8 / 2:00 at RPE 2–3 10:00 at RPE 3–4	**Foundation Run** 5:00 at RPE 2–3 25:00 at RPE 3–4	**Foundation Run** 5:00 at RPE 2–3 25:00 at RPE 3–4
3	Rest	**Hill Repetitions** 5:00 at RPE 2–3 5:00 at RPE 3–4 6 × 0:30* uphill at RPE 8–9 / 1:30 at RPE 2–3 10:00 at RPE 2–3 *Stretch Intervals*	**Foundation Run** 5:00 at RPE 2–3 25:00 at RPE 3–4	**Foundation Run** 5:00 at RPE 2–3 25:00 at RPE 3–4
4	Rest	**VO$_2$max Intervals** 5:00 at RPE 2–3 5:00 at RPE 3–4 4 × 2:00* at RPE 7–8 / 1:00 at RPE 2–3 10:00 at RPE 2–3 *Precision Splitting*	**Foundation Run** 5:00 at RPE 2–3 30:00 at RPE 3–4	**Foundation Run** 5:00 at RPE 2–3 30:00 at RPE 3–4
5	Rest	**Speed Intervals** 5:00 at RPE 2–3 5:00 at RPE 3–4 7 × 1:00* at RPE 8–9 / 2:00 at RPE 2–3 10:00 at RPE 2–3 *Stretch Intervals*	**Foundation Run** 5:00 at RPE 2–3 30:00 at RPE 3–4	**Foundation Run** 5:00 at RPE 2–3 30:00 at RPE 3–4

LEVEL

SSP Steady State Pace
LTP Lactate Threshold Pace
CV Critical Velocity
MAS Maximal Aerobic Speed

FRIDAY	SATURDAY	SUNDAY
Progression Run 5:00 at RPE 2–3 25:00 at RPE 3–4 4:00 at LTP 2:00 at CV 1:00 at MAS 5:00 at RPE 2–3	**Foundation Run** 5:00 at RPE 2–3 25:00 at RPE 3–4	**Endurance Run** 5:00 at RPE 2–3 30:00 at RPE 3–4 5:00 at RPE 5–6
Progression Run 5:00 at RPE 2–3 20:00 at RPE 3–4 8:00 at SSP 4:00 at LTP 2:00 at CV 5:00 at RPE 2–3	**Foundation Run** 5:00 at RPE 2–3 25:00 at RPE 3–4	**Endurance Run** 5:00 at RPE 2–3 40:00 at RPE 3–4 5:00 at RPE 5–6
Fartleks 5:00 at RPE 2–3 5:00 at RPE 3–4 1:00 at CV, 1:00 at RPE 2–3 2:00 at LTP, 1:00 at RPE 2–3 3:00 at SSP, 1:00 at RPE 2–3 2:00 at LTP, 1:00 at RPE 2–3 1:00 at CV, 1:00 at RPE 2–3 10:00 at RPE 3–4	**Foundation Run** 5:00 at RPE 2–3 25:00 at RPE 3–4	**Endurance Run** 5:00 at RPE 2–3 30:00 at RPE 3–4 5:00 at RPE 5–6
Tempo Run 5:00 at RPE 2–3 5:00 at RPE 3–4 10:00 at RPE 6 5:00 at RPE 2–3 10:00 at RPE 6 10:00 at RPE 2–3	**Foundation Run** 5:00 at RPE 2–3 30:00 at RPE 3–4	**Endurance Run** 5:00 at RPE 2–3 50:00 at RPE 3–4 5:00 at RPE 5–6
Critical Velocity Intervals 5:00 at RPE 2–3 5:00 at RPE 3–4 4 × 4:00* at RPE 6–7 / 2:00 at RPE 2–3 10:00 at RPE 2–3 *Precision Splitting*	**Foundation Run** 5:00 at RPE 2–3 30:00 at RPE 3–4	**Endurance Run** 5:00 at RPE 2–3 1:00:00 at RPE 3–4 5:00 at RPE 5–6

	MONDAY	TUESDAY	WEDNESDAY	THURSDAY
6	Rest	**Accelerations** 5:00 at RPE 2–3 5:00 at RPE 3–4 11:00 acceleration 10:00 at RPE 2–3 3:00 acceleration 10:00 at RPE 2–3	**Foundation Run** 5:00 at RPE 2–3 25:00 at RPE 3–4	**Foundation Run** 5:00 at RPE 2–3 25:00 at RPE 3–4
7	Rest	**The Prefontaine** 1 km at RPE 2–3 1 km at RPE 3–4 ? × 200m at RPE 9 / 200m at RPE 6 1 km at RPE 2–3 1 km at RPE 3–4 *(? = Go to failure)*	**Foundation Run** 5:00 at RPE 2–3 35:00 at RPE 3–4	**Foundation Run** 5:00 at RPE 2–3 35:00 at RPE 3–4
8	Rest	**Relaxed Time Trial** 1 km at RPE 2–3 1 km at RPE 3–4 5 km at 95% effort 1:00 rest 2 km at RPE 2–3	**Foundation Run** 5:00 at RPE 2–3 35:00 at RPE 3–4	**Foundation Run** 5:00 at RPE 2–3 35:00 at RPE 3–4
9	Rest	**Fartleks** 5:00 at RPE 2–3 5:00 at RPE 3–4 8 × 1:00 at RPE 7–8 / 2:00 at RPE 2–3 10:00 at RPE 3–4	**Foundation Run** 5:00 at RPE 2–3 30:00 at RPE 3–4	**Fast Finish Run** 5:00 at RPE 2–3 20:00 at RPE 3–4 5:00 at CV

FRIDAY	SATURDAY	SUNDAY
Progression Run 5:00 at RPE 2–3 25:00 at RPE 3–4 4:00 at LTP 2:00 at CV 1:00 at MAS 5:00 at RPE 2–3	**Foundation Run** 5:00 at RPE 2–3 25:00 at RPE 3–4	**Endurance Run** 5:00 at RPE 2–3 40:00 at RPE 3–4 5:00 at RPE 5–6
Tempo Run 5:00 at RPE 2–3 5:00 at RPE 3–4 12:00 at RPE 6 5:00 at RPE 2–3 12:00 at RPE 6 10:00 at RPE 2–3	**Foundation Run** 5:00 at RPE 2–3 35:00 at RPE 3–4	**Endurance Run** 5:00 at RPE 2–3 1:10:00 at RPE 3–4 5:00 at RPE 5–6
Critical Velocity Intervals 5:00 at RPE 2–3 5:00 at RPE 3–4 5 × 4:00* at RPE 6–7 / 2:00 at RPE 2–3 10:00 at RPE 2–3 *Precision Splitting*	**Foundation Run** 5:00 at RPE 2–3 35:00 at RPE 3–4	**Endurance Run** 5:00 at RPE 2–3 50:00 at RPE 3–4 5:00 at RPE 5–6
Foundation Run 5:00 at RPE 2–3 15:00 at RPE 3–4	**5K Race**	Rest

5K

1

5K

This plan is a good fit for experienced competitive runners who are prepared to train hard in pursuit of improved 5K performance. Before starting the plan, be sure to build your training to the point where you're comfortably able to run seven days a week for up to 70 minutes.

	MONDAY	TUESDAY	WEDNESDAY	THURSDAY
1	**Recovery Run** 30:00 at RPE 2–3	**Fartleks** 5:00 at RPE 2–3 10:00 at RPE 3–4 8 × 0:20 at RPE 8–9 / 1:40 at RPE 2–3 15:00 at RPE 3–4	**Foundation Run** 5:00 at RPE 2–3 35:00 at RPE 3–4	**Foundation Run** 5:00 at RPE 2–3 55:00 at RPE 3–4
2	**Recovery Run** 30:00 at RPE 2–3	**Fartleks** 5:00 at RPE 2–3 10:00 at RPE 3–4 8 × 1:00 at RPE 7–8 / 2:00 at RPE 2–3 15:00 at RPE 3–4	**Foundation Run** 5:00 at RPE 2–3 35:00 at RPE 3–4	**Foundation Run** 5:00 at RPE 2–3 55:00 at RPE 3–4
3	Rest	**Hill Repetitions** 5:00 at RPE 2–3 10:00 at RPE 3–4 8 × 0:30* uphill at RPE 8–9 / 1:30 at RPE 2–3 15:00 at RPE 2–3 *Stretch Intervals*	**Foundation Run** 5:00 at RPE 2–3 35:00 at RPE 3–4	**Foundation Run** 5:00 at RPE 2–3 55:00 at RPE 3–4
4	**Recovery Run** 30:00 at RPE 2–3	**VO₂max Intervals** 5:00 at RPE 2–3 10:00 at RPE 3–4 5 × 2:00* at RPE 7–8 / 1:00 at RPE 2–3 15:00 at RPE 2–3 *Precision Splitting*	**Foundation Run** 5:00 at RPE 2–3 40:00 at RPE 3–4	**Foundation Run** 5:00 at RPE 2–3 55:00 at RPE 3–4

LEVEL

SSP Steady State Pace
LTP Lactate Threshold Pace
CV Critical Velocity
MAS Maximal Aerobic Speed

10KP 10K Pace

FRIDAY

Progression Run
5:00 at RPE 2–3
30:00 at RPE 3–4
4:00 at LTP
2:00 at CV
1:00 at MAS
5:00 at RPE 2–3

Progression Run
5:00 at RPE 2–3
30:00 at RPE 3–4
8:00 at SSP
4:00 at LTP
2:00 at CV
5:00 at RPE 2–3

Fartleks
5:00 at RPE 2–3
10:00 at RPE 3–4
1:00 at CV, 1:00 at RPE 2–3
2:00 at LTP, 1:00 at RPE 2–3
3:00 at SSP, 1:00 at RPE 2–3
2:00 at LTP, 1:00 at RPE 2–3
1:00 at CV, 1:00 at RPE 2–3
15:00 at RPE 3–4

Critical Velocity Intervals
5:00 at RPE 2–3
10:00 at RPE 3–4
5 × 4:00* at RPE 6–7 /
  2:00 at RPE 2–3
15:00 at RPE 2–3
*Precision Splitting

SATURDAY

Foundation Run
5:00 at RPE 2–3
35:00 at RPE 3–4

Foundation Run
5:00 at RPE 2–3
35:00 at RPE 3–4

Foundation Run
5:00 at RPE 2–3
35:00 at RPE 3–4

Foundation Run
5:00 at RPE 2–3
40:00 at RPE 3–4

SUNDAY

Endurance Run
5:00 at RPE 2–3
1:00:00 at RPE 3–4
5:00 at RPE 5–6

Steady State Run
5:00 at RPE 2–3
10:00 at RPE 3–4
30:00 at RPE 5
15:00 at RPE 2–3

Endurance Run
5:00 at RPE 2–3
1:10:00 at RPE 3–4
5:00 at RPE 5–6

Tempo Run
5:00 at RPE 2–3
10:00 at RPE 3–4
8:00 at RPE 6
5:00 at RPE 2–3
8:00 at RPE 6
5:00 at RPE 2–3
8:00 at RPE 6
15:00 at RPE 2–3

	MONDAY	TUESDAY	WEDNESDAY	THURSDAY
5	**Recovery Run** 30:00 at RPE 2–3	**Relaxed Time Trial** 1 km at RPE 2–3 2 km at RPE 3–4 5 km at 95% effort 1:00 rest 3 km at RPE 2–3	**Foundation Run** 5:00 at RPE 2–3 40:00 at RPE 3–4	**Foundation Run** 5:00 at RPE 2–3 55:00 at RPE 3–4
6	Rest	**Accelerations** 5:00 at RPE 2–3 10:00 at RPE 3–4 11:00 acceleration 10:00 at RPE 2–3 6:00 acceleration 15:00 at RPE 2–3	**Foundation Run** 5:00 at RPE 2–3 35:00 at RPE 3–4	**Foundation Run** 5:00 at RPE 2–3 55:00 at RPE 3–4
7	**Recovery Run** 30:00 at RPE 2–3	**The Prefontaine** 1 km at RPE 2–3 2.5 km at RPE 3–4 ? × 200m at RPE 9 / 200m at RPE 6 1 km at RPE 2–3 2.5 km at RPE 3–4 *(? = Go to failure)*	**Foundation Run** 5:00 at RPE 2–3 45:00 at RPE 3–4	**Foundation Run** 5:00 at RPE 2–3 55:00 at RPE 3–4
8	**Recovery Run** 30:00 at RPE 2–3	**5K Pace Intervals** 1 km at RPE 2–3 2 km at RPE 3–4 6 × (0.8 km at 10KP / 1:00 rest) 3 km at RPE 2–3	**Foundation Run** 5:00 at RPE 2–3 45:00 at RPE 3–4	**Foundation Run** 5:00 at RPE 2–3 55:00 at RPE 3–4
9	Rest	**Speed Intervals** 5:00 at RPE 2–3 10:00 at RPE 3–4 10 × 0:30* at RPE 8–9 / 1:30 at RPE 2–3 15:00 at RPE 2–3 **Stretch Intervals*	**Foundation Run** 5:00 at RPE 2–3 35:00 at RPE 3–4	**Fast Finish Run** 5:00 at RPE 2–3 25:00 at RPE 3–4 5:00 at CV

FRIDAY	SATURDAY	SUNDAY

Speed Intervals
5:00 at RPE 2–3
10:00 at RPE 3–4
10 × 1:00* at RPE 8–9 /
  2:00 at RPE 2–3
15:00 at RPE 2–3
*Stretch Intervals

Foundation Run
5:00 at RPE 2–3
40:00 at RPE 3–4

Steady State Run
5:00 at RPE 2–3
10:00 at RPE 3–4
35:00 at RPE 5
15:00 at RPE 2–3

Progression Run
5:00 at RPE 2–3
35:00 at RPE 3–4
4:00 at LTP
2:00 at CV
1:00 at MAS
5:00 at RPE 2–3

Foundation Run
5:00 at RPE 2–3
35:00 at RPE 3–4

Endurance Run
5:00 at RPE 2–3
1:20:00 at RPE 3–4
5:00 at RPE 5–6

10K Pace Intervals
1 km at RPE 2–3
2 km at RPE 3–4
8 × (1 km at 10KP / 1:00 rest)
3 km at RPE 2–3

Foundation Run
5:00 at RPE 2–3
45:00 at RPE 3–4

Tempo Run
5:00 at RPE 2–3
10:00 at RPE 3–4
10:00 at RPE 6
5:00 at RPE 2–3
10:00 at RPE 6
5:00 at RPE 2–3
10:00 at RPE 6
15:00 at RPE 2–3

Critical Velocity Intervals
5:00 at RPE 2–3
10:00 at RPE 3–4
6 × 4:00* at RPE 6–7 /
  2:00 at RPE 2–3
15:00 at RPE 2–3
*Precision Splitting

Foundation Run
5:00 at RPE 2–3
45:00 at RPE 3–4

Progression Run
5:00 at RPE 2–3
25:00 at RPE 3–4
16:00 at SSP
8:00 at LTP
4:00 at CV
5:00 at RPE 2–3

Foundation Run
5:00 at RPE 2–3
15:00 at RPE 3–4

5K Race

Rest

5K

This plan is designed for serious, competitive runners seeking the absolute limit of their potential at the 5K distance. Before starting the plan, be sure to build your training to the point where you're comfortably able to run nine times a week for up to 80 minutes.

	MONDAY	TUESDAY	WEDNESDAY	THURSDAY
1	**Recovery Run** 40:00 at RPE 2–3	**Fartleks** 5:00 at RPE 2–3 15:00 at RPE 3–4 10 × 0:20 at RPE 8–9 / 1:40 at RPE 2–3 20:00 at RPE 3–4 **Recovery Run** 20:00 at RPE 2–3	**Foundation Run** 5:00 at RPE 2–3 40:00 at RPE 3–4	**Foundation Run** 5:00 at RPE 2–3 55:00 at RPE 3–4
2	**Recovery Run** 40:00 at RPE 2–3	**Fartleks** 5:00 at RPE 2–3 15:00 at RPE 3–4 10 × 1:00 at RPE 7–8 / 2:00 at RPE 2–3 20:00 at RPE 3–4 **Recovery Run** 20:00 at RPE 2–3	**Foundation Run** 5:00 at RPE 2–3 45:00 at RPE 3–4	**Foundation Run** 5:00 at RPE 2–3 55:00 at RPE 3–4
3	Rest	**Hill Repetitions** 5:00 at RPE 2–3 15:00 at RPE 3–4 10 × 0:30* uphill at RPE 8–9 / 1:30 at RPE 2–3 20:00 at RPE 2–3 *Stretch Intervals* **Recovery Run** 20:00 at RPE 2–3	**Foundation Run** 5:00 at RPE 2–3 40:00 at RPE 3–4	**Foundation Run** 5:00 at RPE 2–3 55:00 at RPE 3–4

LEVEL

SSP Steady State Pace
LTP Lactate Threshold Pace
CV Critical Velocity
MAS Maximal Aerobic Speed

10KP 10K Pace

FRIDAY

Progression Run
5:00 at RPE 2–3
35:00 at RPE 3–4
4:00 at LTP
2:00 at CV
1:00 at MAS
5:00 at RPE 2–3

Recovery Run
20:00 at RPE 2–3

Progression Run
5:00 at RPE 2–3
25:00 at RPE 3–4
12:00 at SSP
6:00 at LTP
3:00 at CV
5:00 at RPE 2–3

Recovery Run
20:00 at RPE 2–3

Fartleks
5:00 at RPE 2–3
15:00 at RPE 3–4
1:00 at CV, 1:00 at RPE 2–3
2:00 at LTP, 1:00 at RPE 2–3
3:00 at SSP, 1:00 at RPE 2–3
2:00 at LTP, 1:00 at RPE 2–3
1:00 at CV, 1:00 at RPE 2–3
2:00 at LTP, 1:00 at RPE 2–3
3:00 at SSP
20:00 at RPE 3–4

Recovery Run
20:00 at RPE 2–3

SATURDAY

Foundation Run
5:00 at RPE 2–3
40:00 at RPE 3–4

Foundation Run
5:00 at RPE 2–3
45:00 at RPE 3–4

Foundation Run
5:00 at RPE 2–3
40:00 at RPE 3–4

SUNDAY

Endurance Run
5:00 at RPE 2–3
1:10:00 at RPE 3–4
5:00 at RPE 5–6

Steady State Run
5:00 at RPE 2–3
15:00 at RPE 3–4
35:00 at RPE 5
20:00 at RPE 2–3

Endurance Run
5:00 at RPE 2–3
1:30:00 at RPE 3–4
5:00 at RPE 5–6

5K

	MONDAY	TUESDAY	WEDNESDAY	THURSDAY
4	**Recovery Run** 40:00 at RPE 2–3	**VO₂max Intervals** 5:00 at RPE 2–3 15:00 at RPE 3–4 6 × 2:00* at RPE 7–8 / 1:00 at RPE 2–3 20:00 at RPE 2–3 *Precision Splitting* **Recovery Run** 25:00 at RPE 2–3	**Foundation Run** 5:00 at RPE 2–3 50:00 at RPE 3–4	**Foundation Run** 5:00 at RPE 2–3 55:00 at RPE 3–4
5	**Recovery Run** 40:00 at RPE 2–3	**Relaxed Time Trial** 1 km at RPE 2–3 3 km at RPE 3–4 5 km at 95% effort 1:00 rest 4 km at RPE 2–3 **Recovery Run** 25:00 at RPE 2–3	**Foundation Run** 5:00 at RPE 2–3 55:00 at RPE 3–4	**Foundation Run** 5:00 at RPE 2–3 55:00 at RPE 3–4
6	Rest	**Accelerations** 5:00 at RPE 2–3 15:00 at RPE 3–4 11:00 acceleration 10:00 at RPE 2–3 6:00 acceleration 20:00 at RPE 2–3 **Recovery Run** 20:00 at RPE 2–3	**Foundation Run** 5:00 at RPE 2–3 45:00 at RPE 3–4	**Foundation Run** 5:00 at RPE 2–3 55:00 at RPE 3–4
7	**Recovery Run** 40:00 at RPE 2–3	**The Prefontaine** 1 km at RPE 2–3 4 km at RPE 3–4 ? × 200m at RPE 9 / 200m at RPE 6 1 km at RPE 2–3 4 km at RPE 3–4 *(? = Go to failure)* **Recovery Run** 30:00 at RPE 2–3	**Foundation Run** 5:00 at RPE 2–3 55:00 at RPE 3–4	**Foundation Run** 5:00 at RPE 2–3 1:00:00 at RPE 3–4
8	**Recovery Run** 40:00 at RPE 2–3	**5K Pace Intervals** 1 km at RPE 2–3 2 km at RPE 3–4 6 × (0.8 km at 10KP / 1:00 rest) 3 km at RPE 2–3 **Recovery Run** 30:00 at RPE 2–3	**Foundation Run** 5:00 at RPE 2–3 55:00 at RPE 3–4	**Foundation Run** 5:00 at RPE 2–3 1:05:00 at RPE 3–4
9	Rest	**Speed Intervals** 5:00 at RPE 2–3 15:00 at RPE 3–4 10 × 0:30* at RPE 8–9 / 1:30 at RPE 2–3 20:00 at RPE 2–3 *Stretch Intervals*	**Foundation Run** 5:00 at RPE 2–3 55:00 at RPE 3–4	**Fast Finish Run** 5:00 at RPE 2–3 30:00 at RPE 3–4 5:00 at CV

FRIDAY	SATURDAY	SUNDAY

Critical Velocity Intervals
5:00 at RPE 2–3
15:00 at RPE 3–4
6 × 4:00* at RPE 6–7 /
  2:00 at RPE 2–3
20:00 at RPE 2–3
*Precision Splitting

Recovery Run
25:00 at RPE 2–3

Foundation Run
5:00 at RPE 2–3
50:00 at RPE 3–4

Tempo Run
5:00 at RPE 2–3
15:00 at RPE 3–4
10:00 at RPE 6
5:00 at RPE 2–3
10:00 at RPE 6
5:00 at RPE 2–3
10:00 at RPE 6
20:00 at RPE 2–3

Speed Intervals
5:00 at RPE 2–3
15:00 at RPE 3–4
12 × 1:00* at RPE 8–9 /
  2:00 at RPE 2–3
20:00 at RPE 2–3
*Stretch Intervals

Recovery Run
25:00 at RPE 2–3

Foundation Run
5:00 at RPE 2–3
55:00 at RPE 3–4

Steady State Run
5:00 at RPE 2–3
15:00 at RPE 3–4
40:00 at RPE 5
20:00 at RPE 2–3

Progression Run
5:00 at RPE 2–3
30:00 at RPE 3–4
8:00 at LTP
4:00 at CV
2:00 at MAS
5:00 at RPE 2–3

Recovery Run
20:00 at RPE 2–3

Foundation Run
5:00 at RPE 2–3
45:00 at RPE 3–4

Endurance Run
5:00 at RPE 2–3
1:50:00 at RPE 3–4
5:00 at RPE 5–6

10K Pace Intervals
1 km at RPE 2–3
3 km at RPE 3–4
8 × (1 km at 10KP / 1:00 rest)
4 km at RPE 2–3

Recovery Run
30:00 at RPE 2–3

Foundation Run
5:00 at RPE 2–3
55:00 at RPE 3–4

Tempo Run
5:00 at RPE 2–3
15:00 at RPE 3–4
12:00 at RPE 6
5:00 at RPE 2–3
12:00 at RPE 6
5:00 at RPE 2–3
12:00 at RPE 6
20:00 at RPE 2–3

Critical Velocity Intervals
5:00 at RPE 2–3
10:00 at RPE 3–4
6 × 4:00* at RPE 6–7 /
  2:00 at RPE 2–3
15:00 at RPE 2–3
*Precision Splitting

Recovery Run
30:00 at RPE 2–3

Foundation Run
5:00 at RPE 2–3
15:00 at RPE 3–4

Foundation Run
5:00 at RPE 2–3
55:00 at RPE 3–4

5K Race

Progression Run
5:00 at RPE 2–3
35:00 at RPE 3–4
16:00 at SSP
8:00 at LTP
4:00 at CV
5:00 at RPE 2–3

Rest

10

10K Training Plans

The four training plans presented in this chapter are designed to help runners master the art of pacing and find their limit at the 10K distance. The various levels cover the needs of everyone from first-timers to elites. Refer back to Chapter 6 for details on the RPE-based intensity scale used throughout the plans and for full explanations of certain terms and workout types. Online versions of the plans are available for separate purchase on the 80/20 Endurance website. Additionally, device-compatible free versions of the individual workouts can be found at 8020endurance.com/on-pace-workouts.

10K

This plan is appropriate for beginning runners preparing for their first 10K event and for more experienced runners who need or prefer a relatively low-volume training program for any reason. Before starting the plan, be sure to build your training to the point where you're comfortably able to run five days a week for up to 40 minutes.

	MONDAY	TUESDAY	WEDNESDAY	THURSDAY
1	Rest	**Fartleks** 5:00 at RPE 2–3 5:00 at RPE 3–4 6 × 0:20 at RPE 8–9 / 1:40 at RPE 2–3 10:00 at RPE 3–4	**Foundation Run** 5:00 at RPE 2–3 20:00 at RPE 3–4	Rest
2	Rest	**Fartleks** 5:00 at RPE 2–3 5:00 at RPE 3–4 6 × 1:00 at RPE 7–8 / 2:00 at RPE 2–3 10:00 at RPE 3–4	**Foundation Run** 5:00 at RPE 2–3 20:00 at RPE 3–4	Rest
3	Rest	**Hill Repetitions** 5:00 at RPE 2–3 5:00 at RPE 3–4 6 × 0:30 uphill at RPE 8–9 / 1:30 at RPE 2–3 10:00 at RPE 2–3	**Foundation Run** 5:00 at RPE 2–3 20:00 at RPE 3–4	Rest
4	Rest	**VO$_2$max Intervals** 5:00 at RPE 2–3 5:00 at RPE 3–4 4 × 2:00 at RPE 7–8 / 1:00 at RPE 2–3 10:00 at RPE 2–3	**Foundation Run** 5:00 at RPE 2–3 25:00 at RPE 3–4	Rest
5	Rest	**Accelerations** 5:00 at RPE 2–3 5:00 at RPE 3–4 11:00 acceleration 10:00 at RPE 2–3 3:00 acceleration 10:00 at RPE 2–3	**Foundation Run** 5:00 at RPE 2–3 25:00 at RPE 3–4	Rest

LEVEL

SSP Steady State Pace
LTP Lactate Threshold Pace
CV Critical Velocity
MAS Maximal Aerobic Speed

5KP 5K Pace
10KP 10K Pace

FRIDAY

Progression Run
5:00 at RPE 2–3
10:00 at RPE 3–4
8:00 at SSP
4:00 at LTP
2:00 at CV
5:00 at RPE 2–3

Progression Run
5:00 at RPE 2–3
20:00 at RPE 3–4
4:00 at LTP
2:00 at CV
1:00 at MAS
5:00 at RPE 2–3

Fartleks
5:00 at RPE 2–3
5:00 at RPE 3–4
1:00 at CV, 1:00 at RPE 2–3
2:00 at LTP, 1:00 at RPE 2–3
3:00 at SSP, 1:00 at RPE 2–3
2:00 at LTP, 1:00 at RPE 2–3
1:00 at CV, 1:00 at RPE 2–3
10:00 at RPE 3–4

Tempo Run
5:00 at RPE 2–3
5:00 at RPE 3–4
10:00 at RPE 6
5:00 at RPE 2–3
10:00 at RPE 6
10:00 at RPE 2–3

Critical Velocity Intervals
5:00 at RPE 2–3
5:00 at RPE 3–4
4 × 4:00 at RPE 6–7 /
   2:00 at RPE 2–3
10:00 at RPE 2–3

SATURDAY

Foundation Run
5:00 at RPE 2–3
20:00 at RPE 3–4

Foundation Run
5:00 at RPE 2–3
20:00 at RPE 3–4

Foundation Run
5:00 at RPE 2–3
20:00 at RPE 3–4

Foundation Run
5:00 at RPE 2–3
25:00 at RPE 3–4

Foundation Run
5:00 at RPE 2–3
25:00 at RPE 3–4

SUNDAY

Endurance Run
5:00 at RPE 2–3
30:00 at RPE 3–4
5:00 at RPE 4–5

Endurance Run
5:00 at RPE 2–3
35:00 at RPE 3–4
5:00 at RPE 4–5

Endurance Run
5:00 at RPE 2–3
30:00 at RPE 3–4
5:00 at RPE 4–5

Endurance Run
5:00 at RPE 2–3
40:00 at RPE 3–4
5:00 at RPE 4–5

Endurance Run
5:00 at RPE 2–3
45:00 at RPE 3–4
5:00 at RPE 4–5

	MONDAY	TUESDAY	WEDNESDAY	THURSDAY
6	Rest	**Hill Repetitions** 5:00 at RPE 2–3 5:00 at RPE 3–4 8 × 0:30 uphill at RPE 8–9 / 1:30 at RPE 2–3 10:00 at RPE 2–3	**Foundation Run** 5:00 at RPE 2–3 25:00 at RPE 3–4	Rest
7	Rest	**5K Pace Intervals** 1 km at RPE 2–3 1 km at RPE 3–4 8 × (0.6 km at 5KP / 1:00 rest) 2 km at RPE 2–3	**Foundation Run** 5:00 at RPE 2–3 30:00 at RPE 3–4	Rest
8	Rest	**Speed Intervals** 5:00 at RPE 2–3 5:00 at RPE 3–4 8 × 0:45 at RPE 8–9 / 1:45 at RPE 2–3 10:00 at RPE 2–3	**Foundation Run** 5:00 at RPE 2–3 30:00 at RPE 3–4	Rest
9	Rest	**Accelerations** 5:00 at RPE 2–3 5:00 at RPE 3–4 11:00 acceleration 10:00 at RPE 2–3 6:00 acceleration 10:00 at RPE 2–3	**Foundation Run** 5:00 at RPE 2–3 30:00 at RPE 3–4	Rest
10	Rest	**VO$_2$max Intervals** 5:00 at RPE 2–3 5:00 at RPE 3–4 5 × 2:00 at RPE 7–8 / 1:00 at RPE 2–3 10:00 at RPE 2–3	**Foundation Run** 5:00 at RPE 2–3 35:00 at RPE 3–4	Rest
11	Rest	**5K Pace Intervals** 1 km at RPE 2–3 1 km at RPE 3–4 6 × (0.8 km at 5KP / 1:00 rest) 2 km at RPE 2–3	**Foundation Run** 5:00 at RPE 2–3 35:00 at RPE 3–4	Rest
12	Rest	**Fartleks** 5:00 at RPE 2–3 5:00 at RPE 3–4 6 × 1:00 at RPE 7–8 / 2:00 at RPE 2–3 10:00 at RPE 3–4	Rest	**Fast Finish Run** 5:00 at RPE 2–3 10:00 at RPE 3–4 5:00 at RPE 6–7

FRIDAY	SATURDAY	SUNDAY
Progression Run 5:00 at RPE 2–3 10:00 at RPE 3–4 12:00 at SSP 6:00 at LTP 3:00 at CV 5:00 at RPE 2–3	**Foundation Run** 5:00 at RPE 2–3 25:00 at RPE 3–4	**Endurance Run** 5:00 at RPE 2–3 35:00 at RPE 3–4 5:00 at RPE 4–5
Steady State Run 5:00 at RPE 2–3 5:00 at RPE 3–4 25:00 at RPE 5 10:00 at RPE 2–3	**Foundation Run** 5:00 at RPE 2–3 30:00 at RPE 3–4	**Endurance Run** 5:00 at RPE 2–3 50:00 at RPE 3–4 5:00 at RPE 4–5
Tempo Run 5:00 at RPE 2–3 5:00 at RPE 3–4 12:00 at RPE 6 5:00 at RPE 2–3 12:00 at RPE 6 10:00 at RPE 2–3	**Foundation Run** 5:00 at RPE 2–3 30:00 at RPE 3–4	**Endurance Run** 5:00 at RPE 2–3 1:00:00 at RPE 3–4 5:00 at RPE 4–5
Fartleks 5:00 at RPE 2–3 5:00 at RPE 3–4 1:00 at CV, 1:00 at RPE 2–3 2:00 at LTP, 1:00 at RPE 2–3 3:00 at SSP, 1:00 at RPE 2–3 2:00 at LTP, 1:00 at RPE 2–3 1:00 at CV, 1:00 at RPE 2–3 2:00 at LTP, 1:00 at RPE 2–3 3:00 at SSP, 1:00 at RPE 2–3 10:00 at RPE 3–4	**Foundation Run** 5:00 at RPE 2–3 30:00 at RPE 3–4	**Endurance Run** 5:00 at RPE 2–3 40:00 at RPE 3–4 5:00 at RPE 4–5
Critical Velocity Intervals 5:00 at RPE 2–3 5:00 at RPE 3–4 5 × 4:00 at RPE 6–7 / 2:00 at RPE 2–3 10:00 at RPE 2–3	**Foundation Run** 5:00 at RPE 2–3 35:00 at RPE 3–4	**Endurance Run** 5:00 at RPE 2–3 1:10:00 at RPE 3–4 5:00 at RPE 4–5
Fartleks 5:00 at RPE 2–3 5:00 at RPE 3–4 6 × 2:00 at RPE 6 / 2:00 at RPE 2–3 10:00 at RPE 3–4	**Foundation Run** 5:00 at RPE 2–3 35:00 at RPE 3–4	**10K Pace Intervals** 1 km at RPE 2–3 2 km at RPE 3–4 8 × (1 km at 10KP / 1:00 rest) 3 km at RPE 2–3
Foundation Run 5:00 at RPE 2–3 15:00 at RPE 3–4	**10K Race**	Rest

10K

This plan is designed for runners who are ready to take their training load up a notch in order to improve their 10K time. Before starting the plan, be sure to build your training to the point where you're comfortably able to run six days a week for up to 40 minutes.

	MONDAY	TUESDAY	WEDNESDAY	THURSDAY
1	Rest	**Fartleks** 5:00 at RPE 2–3 5:00 at RPE 3–4 8 × 0:20 at RPE 8–9 / 1:40 at RPE 2–3 10:00 at RPE 3–4	**Foundation Run** 5:00 at RPE 2–3 25:00 at RPE 3–4	**Foundation Run** 5:00 at RPE 2–3 25:00 at RPE 3–4
2	Rest	**Fartleks** 5:00 at RPE 2–3 5:00 at RPE 3–4 8 × 1:00 at RPE 7–8 / 2:00 at RPE 2–3 10:00 at RPE 3–4	**Foundation Run** 5:00 at RPE 2–3 25:00 at RPE 3–4	**Foundation Run** 5:00 at RPE 2–3 25:00 at RPE 3–4
3	Rest	**Hill Repetitions** 5:00 at RPE 2–3 5:00 at RPE 3–4 8 × 0:30 uphill at RPE 8–9 / 1:30 at RPE 2–3 10:00 at RPE 2–3	**Foundation Run** 5:00 at RPE 2–3 25:00 at RPE 3–4	**Foundation Run** 5:00 at RPE 2–3 25:00 at RPE 3–4
4	Rest	**VO$_2$max Intervals** 5:00 at RPE 2–3 5:00 at RPE 3–4 5 × 2:00 at RPE 7–8 / 1:00 at RPE 2–3 10:00 at RPE 2–3	**Foundation Run** 5:00 at RPE 2–3 30:00 at RPE 3–4	**Foundation Run** 5:00 at RPE 2–3 30:00 at RPE 3–4
5	Rest	**Accelerations** 5:00 at RPE 2–3 5:00 at RPE 3–4 11:00 acceleration 10:00 at RPE 2–3 3:00 acceleration 10:00 at RPE 2–3	**Foundation Run** 5:00 at RPE 2–3 30:00 at RPE 3–4	**Foundation Run** 5:00 at RPE 2–3 30:00 at RPE 3–4

LEVEL

SSP   Steady State Pace
LTP   Lactate Threshold Pace
CV   Critical Velocity
MAS Maximal Aerobic Speed

5KP   5K Pace
10KP 10K Pace
HMP Half-Marathon Pace

FRIDAY	SATURDAY	SUNDAY
Progression Run 5:00 at RPE 2–3 15:00 at RPE 3–4 8:00 at SSP 4:00 at LTP 2:00 at CV 5:00 at RPE 2–3	**Foundation Run** 5:00 at RPE 2–3 25:00 at RPE 3–4	**Endurance Run** 5:00 at RPE 2–3 30:00 at RPE 3–4 5:00 at RPE 4–5
Progression Run 5:00 at RPE 2–3 25:00 at RPE 3–4 4:00 at LTP 2:00 at CV 1:00 at MAS 5:00 at RPE 2–3	**Foundation Run** 5:00 at RPE 2–3 25:00 at RPE 3–4	**Endurance Run** 5:00 at RPE 2–3 40:00 at RPE 3–4 5:00 at RPE 4–5

Progression Fartleks
5:00 at RPE 2–3
5:00 at RPE 3–4
2 × (3:00 at RPE 4–5 /
  1:00 at RPE 2–3)
2 × (4:00 at RPE 5–6 /
  1:00 at RPE 2–3)
10:00 at RPE 2–3
	Foundation Run
	5:00 at RPE 2–3
	25:00 at RPE 3–4
		Endurance Run
		5:00 at RPE 2–3
		30:00 at RPE 3–4
		5:00 at RPE 4–5

Tempo Run 5:00 at RPE 2–3 5:00 at RPE 3–4 12:00 at RPE 6 5:00 at RPE 2–3 12:00 at RPE 6 10:00 at RPE 2–3	**Foundation Run** 5:00 at RPE 2–3 30:00 at RPE 3–4	**Endurance Run** 5:00 at RPE 2–3 50:00 at RPE 3–4 5:00 at RPE 4–5
Critical Velocity Intervals 5:00 at RPE 2–3 5:00 at RPE 3–4 5 × 4:00 at RPE 6–7 / 2:00 at RPE 2–3 10:00 at RPE 2–3	**Foundation Run** 5:00 at RPE 2–3 30:00 at RPE 3–4	**Endurance Run** 5:00 at RPE 2–3 1:00:00 at RPE 3–4 5:00 at RPE 4–5

	MONDAY	TUESDAY	WEDNESDAY	THURSDAY
6	Rest	**Hill Repetitions** 5:00 at RPE 2–3 5:00 at RPE 3–4 6 × 1:00 uphill at RPE 8–9 / 2:00 at RPE 2–3 10:00 at RPE 2–3	**Foundation Run** 5:00 at RPE 2–3 30:00 at RPE 3–4	**Foundation Run** 5:00 at RPE 2–3 30:00 at RPE 3–4
7	Rest	**5K Pace Intervals** 1 km at RPE 2–3 1 km at RPE 3–4 8 × (0.6 km at 5KP / 1:00 rest) 2 km at RPE 2–3	**Foundation Run** 5:00 at RPE 2–3 35:00 at RPE 3–4	**Foundation Run** 5:00 at RPE 2–3 35:00 at RPE 3–4
8	Rest	**Speed Intervals** 5:00 at RPE 2–3 5:00 at RPE 3–4 8 × 1:00 at RPE 8–9 / 2:00 at RPE 2–3 10:00 at RPE 2–3	**Foundation Run** 5:00 at RPE 2–3 35:00 at RPE 3–4	**Foundation Run** 5:00 at RPE 2–3 35:00 at RPE 3–4
9	Rest	**Accelerations** 5:00 at RPE 2–3 5:00 at RPE 3–4 11:00 acceleration 10:00 at RPE 2–3 6:00 acceleration 10:00 at RPE 2–3	**Foundation Run** 5:00 at RPE 2–3 30:00 at RPE 3–4	**Foundation Run** 5:00 at RPE 2–3 30:00 at RPE 3–4
10	Rest	**The Prefontaine** 1 km at RPE 2–3 1 km at RPE 3–4 ? × 200m at RPE 9 / 200m at RPE 6 1 km at RPE 2–3 1 km at RPE 3–4 *(? = Go to failure)*	**Foundation Run** 5:00 at RPE 2–3 40:00 at RPE 3–4	**Foundation Run** 5:00 at RPE 2–3 40:00 at RPE 3–4
11	Rest	**5K Pace Intervals** 1 km at RPE 2–3 1 km at RPE 3–4 6 × (0.8 km at 5KP / 1:00 rest) 2 km at RPE 2–3	**Foundation Run** 5:00 at RPE 2–3 40:00 at RPE 3–4	**Foundation Run** 5:00 at RPE 2–3 40:00 at RPE 3–4
12	Rest	**Fartleks** 5:00 at RPE 2–3 5:00 at RPE 3–4 8 × 1:00 at RPE 7–8 / 2:00 at RPE 2–3 10:00 at RPE 3–4	**Foundation Run** 5:00 at RPE 2–3 30:00 at RPE 3–4	**Fast Finish Run** 5:00 at RPE 2–3 25:00 at RPE 3–4 5:00 at RPE 6–7

FRIDAY	SATURDAY	SUNDAY
Progression Run 5:00 at RPE 2–3 20:00 at RPE 3–4 12:00 at SSP 6:00 at LTP 3:00 at CV 5:00 at RPE 2–3	**Foundation Run** 5:00 at RPE 2–3 30:00 at RPE 3–4	**Endurance Run** 5:00 at RPE 2–3 40:00 at RPE 3–4 5:00 at RPE 4–5
Steady State Run 5:00 at RPE 2–3 5:00 at RPE 3–4 30:00 at RPE 5 10:00 at RPE 2–3	**Foundation Run** 5:00 at RPE 2–3 35:00 at RPE 3–4	**Endurance Run** 5:00 at RPE 2–3 1:10:00 at RPE 3–4 5:00 at RPE 4–5
Tempo Run 5:00 at RPE 2–3 5:00 at RPE 3–4 14:00 at RPE 6 5:00 at RPE 2–3 14:00 at RPE 6 10:00 at RPE 2–3	**Foundation Run** 5:00 at RPE 2–3 35:00 at RPE 3–4	**Endurance Run** 5:00 at RPE 2–3 1:10:00 at RPE 3–4 5:00 at RPE 4–5

Progression Fartleks
5:00 at RPE 2–3
5:00 at RPE 3–4
2 × (3:00 at RPE 4–5 /
   1:00 at RPE 2–3)
2 × (4:00 at RPE 5–6 /
   1:00 at RPE 2–3)
2 × (5:00 at RPE 6–7 /
   1:00 at RPE 2–3)
10:00 at RPE 2–3
	Foundation Run
	5:00 at RPE 2–3
	30:00 at RPE 3–4
		Endurance Run
		5:00 at RPE 2–3
		1:00:00 at RPE 3–4
		5:00 at RPE 4–5

Critical Velocity Intervals 5:00 at RPE 2–3 5:00 at RPE 3–4 6 × 4:00 at RPE 6–7 / 2:00 at RPE 2–3 10:00 at RPE 2–3	**Foundation Run** 5:00 at RPE 2–3 40:00 at RPE 3–4	**Half-Marathon Pace Run** 1 km at RPE 2–3 1 km at RPE 3–4 3 × (3 km at HMP / 1:00 rest) 2 km at RPE 2–3
10K Pace Intervals 1 km at RPE 2–3 1 km at RPE 3–4 8 × (1 km at 10KP / 1:00 rest) 2 km at RPE 2–3	**Foundation Run** 5:00 at RPE 2–3 40:00 at RPE 3–4	**Endurance Run** 5:00 at RPE 2–3 1:00:00 at RPE 3–4 5:00 at RPE 4–5
Foundation Run 5:00 at RPE 2–3 15:00 at RPE 3–4	**10K Race**	Rest

10K

1

10K

This plan is a good fit for experienced competitive runners who are prepared to train hard in pursuit of improved 10K performance. Before starting the plan, be sure to build your training to the point where you're comfortably able to run seven days a week for up to 70 minutes.

	MONDAY	TUESDAY	WEDNESDAY	THURSDAY
1	**Recovery Run** 30:00 at RPE 2–3	**Fartleks** 5:00 at RPE 2–3 10:00 at RPE 3–4 8 × 0:20 at RPE 8–9 / 1:40 at RPE 2–3 15:00 at RPE 3–4	**Foundation Run** 5:00 at RPE 2–3 40:00 at RPE 3–4	**Foundation Run** 5:00 at RPE 2–3 40:00 at RPE 3–4
2	**Recovery Run** 30:00 at RPE 2–3	**Fartleks** 5:00 at RPE 2–3 10:00 at RPE 3–4 8 × 1:00 at RPE 7–8 / 2:00 at RPE 2–3 15:00 at RPE 3–4	**Foundation Run** 5:00 at RPE 2–3 40:00 at RPE 3–4	**Foundation Run** 5:00 at RPE 2–3 40:00 at RPE 3–4
3	Rest	**Hill Repetitions** 5:00 at RPE 2–3 10:00 at RPE 3–4 8 × 0:30 uphill at RPE 8–9 / 1:30 at RPE 2–3 15:00 at RPE 2–3	**Foundation Run** 5:00 at RPE 2–3 40:00 at RPE 3–4	**Foundation Run** 5:00 at RPE 2–3 40:00 at RPE 3–4
4	**Recovery Run** 30:00 at RPE 2–3	**VO₂max Intervals** 5:00 at RPE 2–3 10:00 at RPE 3–4 6 × 2:00 at RPE 7–8 / 1:00 at RPE 2–3 15:00 at RPE 2–3	**Foundation Run** 5:00 at RPE 2–3 45:00 at RPE 3–4	**Foundation Run** 5:00 at RPE 2–3 45:00 at RPE 3–4
5	**Recovery Run** 30:00 at RPE 2–3	**Accelerations** 5:00 at RPE 2–3 10:00 at RPE 3–4 11:00 acceleration 10:00 at RPE 2–3 6:00 acceleration 15:00 at RPE 2–3	**Foundation Run** 5:00 at RPE 2–3 45:00 at RPE 3–4	**Foundation Run** 5:00 at RPE 2–3 45:00 at RPE 3–4

LEVEL

SSP Steady State Pace
LTP Lactate Threshold Pace
CV Critical Velocity
MAS Maximal Aerobic Speed

5KP 5K Pace
10KP 10K Pace
HMP Half-Marathon Pace

FRIDAY	SATURDAY	SUNDAY
Progression Run 5:00 at RPE 2–3 25:00 at RPE 3–4 8:00 at SSP 4:00 at LTP 2:00 at CV 5:00 at RPE 2–3	**Foundation Run** 5:00 at RPE 2–3 40:00 at RPE 3–4	**Endurance Run** 5:00 at RPE 2–3 1:00:00 at RPE 3–4 5:00 at RPE 4–5
Progression Run 5:00 at RPE 2–3 35:00 at RPE 3–4 4:00 at LTP 2:00 at CV 1:00 at MAS 5:00 at RPE 2–3	**Foundation Run** 5:00 at RPE 2–3 40:00 at RPE 3–4	**Endurance Run** 5:00 at RPE 2–3 1:10:00 at RPE 3–4 5:00 at RPE 4–5
Fartleks 5:00 at RPE 2–3 10:00 at RPE 3–4 1:00 at CV, 1:00 at RPE 2–3 2:00 at LTP, 1:00 at RPE 2–3 3:00 at SSP, 1:00 at RPE 2–3 2:00 at LTP, 1:00 at RPE 2–3 1:00 at CV, 1:00 at RPE 2–3 2:00 at LTP, 1:00 at RPE 2–3 3:00 at SSP, 1:00 at RPE 2–3 15:00 at RPE 3–4	**Foundation Run** 5:00 at RPE 2–3 40:00 at RPE 3–4	**Endurance Run** 5:00 at RPE 2–3 1:00:00 at RPE 3–4 5:00 at RPE 4–5
Critical Velocity Intervals 5:00 at RPE 2–3 10:00 at RPE 3–4 6 × 4:00 at RPE 6–7 / 2:00 at RPE 2–3 15:00 at RPE 2–3	**Foundation Run** 5:00 at RPE 2–3 45:00 at RPE 3–4	**Steady State Run** 5:00 at RPE 2–3 10:00 at RPE 3–4 30:00 at RPE 5 15:00 at RPE 2–3

10K Pace Intervals
1 km at RPE 2–3
2 km at RPE 3–4
8 × (1 km at 10KP / 1:00 rest)
3 km at RPE 2–3
	Foundation Run
	5:00 at RPE 2–3
	45:00 at RPE 3–4
		Progression Fartleks
		5:00 at RPE 2–3
		10:00 at RPE 3–4
		2 × (3:00 at RPE 4–5 /
		  1:00 at RPE 2–3)
		2 × (4:00 at RPE 5–6 /
		  1:00 at RPE 2–3)
		2 × (5:00 at RPE 6–7 /
		  1:00 at RPE 2–3)
		15:00 at RPE 2–3

10K

2

	MONDAY	TUESDAY	WEDNESDAY	THURSDAY
6	Rest	**Speed Intervals** 5:00 at RPE 2–3 10:00 at RPE 3–4 8 × 1:00 at RPE 8–9 / 2:00 at RPE 2–3 15:00 at RPE 2–3	**Foundation Run** 5:00 at RPE 2–3 45:00 at RPE 3–4	**Foundation Run** 5:00 at RPE 2–3 45:00 at RPE 3–4
7	**Recovery Run** 30:00 at RPE 2–3	**5K Pace Intervals** 1 km at RPE 2–3 2 km at RPE 3–4 8 × (0.6 km at 5KP / 1:00 rest) 3 km at RPE 2–3	**Foundation Run** 5:00 at RPE 2–3 50:00 at RPE 3–4	**Foundation Run** 5:00 at RPE 2–3 50:00 at RPE 3–4
8	**Recovery Run** 30:00 at RPE 2–3	**Hill Repetitions** 5:00 at RPE 2–3 10:00 at RPE 3–4 10 × 1:00 uphill at RPE 8–9 / 2:00 at RPE 2–3 15:00 at RPE 2–3	**Foundation Run** 5:00 at RPE 2–3 50:00 at RPE 3–4	**Foundation Run** 5:00 at RPE 2–3 50:00 at RPE 3–4
9	Rest	**Accelerations** 5:00 at RPE 2–3 5:00 at RPE 3–4 11:00 acceleration 10:00 at RPE 2–3 6:00 acceleration 10:00 at RPE 2–3 3:00 acceleration 10:00 at RPE 2–3	**Foundation Run** 5:00 at RPE 2–3 50:00 at RPE 3–4	**Foundation Run** 5:00 at RPE 2–3 50:00 at RPE 3–4
10	**Recovery Run** 30:00 at RPE 2–3	**The Prefontaine** 1 km at RPE 2–3 2.5 km at RPE 3–4 ? × 200m at RPE 9 / 200m at RPE 6 1 km at RPE 2–3 2.5 km at RPE 3–4 *(? = Go to failure)*	**Foundation Run** 5:00 at RPE 2–3 55:00 at RPE 3–4	**Foundation Run** 5:00 at RPE 2–3 55:00 at RPE 3–4
11	**Recovery Run** 30:00 at RPE 2–3	**5K Pace Intervals** 1 km at RPE 2–3 2 km at RPE 3–4 6 × (0.8 km at 5KP / 1:00 rest) 3 km at RPE 2–3	**Foundation Run** 5:00 at RPE 2–3 55:00 at RPE 3–4	**Foundation Run** 5:00 at RPE 2–3 50:00 at RPE 3–4
12	Rest	**Fartleks** 5:00 at RPE 2–3 10:00 at RPE 3–4 8 × 1:00 at RPE 7–8 / 2:00 at RPE 2–3 15:00 at RPE 3–4	**Foundation Run** 5:00 at RPE 2–3 40:00 at RPE 3–4	**Fast Finish Run** 5:00 at RPE 2–3 25:00 at RPE 3–4 5:00 at RPE 6–7

FRIDAY	SATURDAY	SUNDAY
Progression Run 5:00 at RPE 2–3 20:00 at RPE 3–4 12:00 at SSP 6:00 at LTP 3:00 at CV 5:00 at RPE 2–3	**Foundation Run** 5:00 at RPE 2–3 45:00 at RPE 3–4	**Endurance Run** 5:00 at RPE 2–3 1:20:00 at RPE 3–4 5:00 at RPE 4–5
Half-Marathon Pace Run 1 km at RPE 2–3 2 km at RPE 3–4 3 × (3 km at HMP / 1:00 rest) 3 km at RPE 2–3	**Foundation Run** 5:00 at RPE 2–3 50:00 at RPE 3–4	**Tempo Run** 5:00 at RPE 2–3 10:00 at RPE 3–4 10:00 at RPE 6, 5:00 at RPE 2–3 10:00 at RPE 6, 5:00 at RPE 2–3 10:00 at RPE 6, 5:00 at RPE 2–3 15:00 at RPE 2–3
Critical Velocity Intervals 5:00 at RPE 2–3 10:00 at RPE 3–4 7 × 4:00 at RPE 6–7 / 2:00 at RPE 2–3 15:00 at RPE 2–3	**Foundation Run** 5:00 at RPE 2–3 50:00 at RPE 3–4	**Steady State Run** 5:00 at RPE 2–3 10:00 at RPE 3–4 40:00 at RPE 5 15:00 at RPE 2–3
Fartleks 5:00 at RPE 2–3 10:00 at RPE 3–4 1:00 at CV, 1:00 at RPE 2–3 2:00 at LTP, 1:00 at RPE 2–3 3:00 at SSP, 1:00 at RPE 2–3 2:00 at LTP, 1:00 at RPE 2–3 1:00 at CV, 1:00 at RPE 2–3 2:00 at LTP, 1:00 at RPE 2–3 3:00 at SSP, 1:00 at RPE 2–3 15:00 at RPE 3–4	**Foundation Run** 5:00 at RPE 2–3 50:00 at RPE 3–4	**Endurance Run** 5:00 at RPE 2–3 1:30:00 at RPE 3–4 5:00 at RPE 4–5

10K Relaxed Time Trial
1 km at RPE 2–3
2 km at RPE 3–4
10 km at 95% effort
3 km at RPE 2–3
	Foundation Run
	5:00 at RPE 2–3
	55:00 at RPE 3–4
		Progression Fartleks
		5:00 at RPE 2–3
		10:00 at RPE 3–4
		2 × (3:00 at RPE 4–5 /
		    1:00 at RPE 2–3)
		2 × (4:00 at RPE 5–6 /
		    1:00 at RPE 2–3)
		2 × (5:00 at RPE 6–7 /
		    1:00 at RPE 2–3)
		2 × (6:00 at RPE 7–8 /
		    1:00 at RPE 2–3)
		15:00 at RPE 2–3

10K Pace Intervals 1 km at RPE 2–3 2 km at RPE 3–4 10 × (1 km at 10KP / 1:00 rest) 3 km at RPE 2–3	**Foundation Run** 5:00 at RPE 2–3 45:00 at RPE 3–4	**Endurance Run** 5:00 at RPE 2–3 1:00:00 at RPE 3–4 5:00 at RPE 4–5
Foundation Run 5:00 at RPE 2–3 15:00 at RPE 3–4	**10K Race**	Rest

2 10K

10K

This plan is designed for serious, competitive runners seeking the absolute limit of their potential at the 10K distance. Before starting the plan, be sure to build your training to the point where you're comfortably able to run nine times per week for up to 80 minutes.

	MONDAY	TUESDAY	WEDNESDAY	THURSDAY
1	**Recovery Run** 40:00 at RPE 2–3	**Fartleks** 5:00 at RPE 2–3 15:00 at RPE 3–4 10 × 0:20 at RPE 8–9 / 1:40 at RPE 2–3 20:00 at RPE 3–4 **Recovery Run** 20:00 at RPE 2–3	**Foundation Run** 5:00 at RPE 2–3 55:00 at RPE 3–4	**Foundation Run** 5:00 at RPE 2–3 55:00 at RPE 3–4
2	**Recovery Run** 40:00 at RPE 2–3	**Fartleks** 5:00 at RPE 2–3 15:00 at RPE 3–4 10 × 1:00 at RPE 7–8 / 2:00 at RPE 2–3 20:00 at RPE 3–4 **Recovery Run** 20:00 at RPE 2–3	**Foundation Run** 5:00 at RPE 2–3 55:00 at RPE 3–4	**Foundation Run** 5:00 at RPE 2–3 55:00 at RPE 3–4
3	Rest	**Hill Repetitions** 5:00 at RPE 2–3 15:00 at RPE 3–4 10 × 0:30 uphill at RPE 8–9 / 1:30 at RPE 2–3 20:00 at RPE 3–4 **Recovery Run** 20:00 at RPE 2–3	**Foundation Run** 5:00 at RPE 2–3 45:00 at RPE 3–4	**Foundation Run** 5:00 at RPE 2–3 50:00 at RPE 3–4

LEVEL

SSP Steady State Pace
LTP Lactate Threshold Pace
CV Critical Velocity
MAS Maximal Aerobic Speed

5KP 5K Pace
10KP 10K Pace
HMP Half-Marathon Pace

FRIDAY	SATURDAY	SUNDAY
Progression Run 5:00 at RPE 2–3 35:00 at RPE 3–4 8:00 at SSP 4:00 at LTP 2:00 at CV 5:00 at RPE 2–3 **Recovery Run** 20:00 at RPE 2–3	**Foundation Run** 5:00 at RPE 2–3 55:00 at RPE 3–4	**Endurance Run** 5:00 at RPE 2–3 1:10:00 at RPE 3–4 5:00 at RPE 4–5
Progression Run 5:00 at RPE 2–3 35:00 at RPE 3–4 8:00 at LTP 4:00 at CV 2:00 at MAS 5:00 at RPE 2–3 **Recovery Run** 20:00 at RPE 2–3	**Foundation Run** 5:00 at RPE 2–3 55:00 at RPE 3–4	**Endurance Run** 5:00 at RPE 2–3 1:30:00 at RPE 3–4 5:00 at RPE 4–5
Fartleks 5:00 at RPE 2–3 15:00 at RPE 3–4 1:00 at CV, 1:00 at RPE 2–3 2:00 at LTP, 1:00 at RPE 2–3 3:00 at SSP, 1:00 at RPE 2–3 2:00 at LTP, 1:00 at RPE 2–3 1:00 at CV, 1:00 at RPE 2–3 2:00 at LTP, 1:00 at RPE 2–3 3:00 at SSP, 1:00 at RPE 2–3 2:00 at LTP, 1:00 at RPE 2–3 1:00 at CV, 1:00 at RPE 2–3 20:00 at RPE 3–4 **Recovery Run** 20:00 at RPE 2–3	**Foundation Run** 5:00 at RPE 2–3 45:00 at RPE 3–4	**Endurance Run** 5:00 at RPE 2–3 1:10:00 at RPE 3–4 5:00 at RPE 4–5

	MONDAY	TUESDAY	WEDNESDAY	THURSDAY
4	**Recovery Run** 40:00 at RPE 2–3	**VO₂max Intervals** 5:00 at RPE 2–3 15:00 at RPE 3–4 7 × 2:00 at RPE 7–8 / 1:00 at RPE 2–3 20:00 at RPE 2–3 **Recovery Run** 25:00 at RPE 2–3	**Foundation Run** 5:00 at RPE 2–3 55:00 at RPE 3–4	**Foundation Run** 5:00 at RPE 2–3 1:00:00 at RPE 3–4
5	**Recovery Run** 40:00 at RPE 2–3	**Accelerations** 5:00 at RPE 2–3 15:00 at RPE 3–4 11:00 acceleration 10:00 at RPE 2–3 6:00 acceleration 3:00 acceleration 20:00 at RPE 2–3 **Recovery Run** 25:00 at RPE 2–3	**Foundation Run** 5:00 at RPE 2–3 55:00 at RPE 3–4	**Foundation Run** 5:00 at RPE 2–3 1:00:00 at RPE 3–4
6	Rest	**Speed Intervals** 5:00 at RPE 2–3 15:00 at RPE 3–4 8 × 0:45 at RPE 8–9 / 1:45 at RPE 2–3 20:00 at RPE 2–3 **Recovery Run** 20:00 at RPE 2–3	**Foundation Run** 5:00 at RPE 2–3 50:00 at RPE 3–4	**Foundation Run** 5:00 at RPE 2–3 55:00 at RPE 3–4
7	**Recovery Run** 40:00 at RPE 2–3	**5K Pace Intervals** 1 km at RPE 2–3 3 km at RPE 3–4 8 × (0.6 km at 5KP / 1:00 rest) 4 km at RPE 2–3 **Recovery Run** 30:00 at RPE 2–3	**Foundation Run** 5:00 at RPE 2–3 55:00 at RPE 3–4	**Foundation Run** 5:00 at RPE 2–3 1:05:00 at RPE 3–4
8	**Recovery Run** 40:00 at RPE 2–3	**Hill Repetitions** 5:00 at RPE 2–3 15:00 at RPE 3–4 12 × 1:00 uphill at RPE 8–9 / 2:00 at RPE 2–3 20:00 at RPE 2–3 **Recovery Run** 30:00 at RPE 2–3	**Foundation Run** 5:00 at RPE 2–3 55:00 at RPE 3–4	**Foundation Run** 5:00 at RPE 2–3 1:05:00 at RPE 3–4

FRIDAY	SATURDAY	SUNDAY
Critical Velocity Intervals 5:00 at RPE 2–3 15:00 at RPE 3–4 7 × 4:00 at RPE 6–7 / 2:00 at RPE 2–3 20:00 at RPE 2–3 **Recovery Run** 25:00 at RPE 2–3	**Foundation Run** 5:00 at RPE 2–3 55:00 at RPE 3–4	**Steady State Run** 5:00 at RPE 2–3 15:00 at RPE 3–4 40:00 at RPE 5 20:00 at RPE 2–3

10K Pace Intervals
1 km at RPE 2–3
3 km at RPE 3–4
8 × (1 km at 10KP / 1:00 rest)
4 km at RPE 2–3
 	
Recovery Run
25:00 at RPE 2–3
	Foundation Run
	5:00 at RPE 2–3
	55:00 at RPE 3–4
		Progression Fartleks
		5:00 at RPE 2–3
		15:00 at RPE 3–4
		2 × (3:00 at RPE 4–5 /
		  1:00 at RPE 2–3)
		2 × (4:00 at RPE 5–6 /
		  1:00 at RPE 2–3)
		2 × (5:00 at RPE 6–7 /
		  1:00 at RPE 2–3)
		20:00 at RPE 2–3

Progression Run 5:00 at RPE 2–3 30:00 at RPE 3–4 12:00 at SSP 6:00 at LTP 3:00 at CV 5:00 at RPE 2–3 **Recovery Run** 20:00 at RPE 2–3	**Foundation Run** 5:00 at RPE 2–3 50:00 at RPE 3–4	**Endurance Run** 5:00 at RPE 2–3 1:30:00 at RPE 3–4 5:00 at RPE 4–5
Half-Marathon Pace Run 1 km at RPE 2–3 3 km at RPE 3–4 3 × (3 km at HMP / 1:00 rest) 4 km at RPE 2–3 **Recovery Run** 30:00 at RPE 2–3	**Foundation Run** 5:00 at RPE 2–3 55:00 at RPE 3–4	**Tempo Run** 5:00 at RPE 2–3 15:00 at RPE 3–4 10:00 at RPE 6, 5:00 at RPE 2–3 10:00 at RPE 6, 5:00 at RPE 2–3 10:00 at RPE 6, 5:00 at RPE 2–3 20:00 at RPE 2–3
Critical Velocity Intervals 5:00 at RPE 2–3 15:00 at RPE 3–4 8 × 4:00 at RPE 6–7 / 2:00 at RPE 2–3 15:00 at RPE 2–3 **Recovery Run** 30:00 at RPE 2–3	**Foundation Run** 5:00 at RPE 2–3 55:00 at RPE 3–4	**Steady State Run** 5:00 at RPE 2–3 15:00 at RPE 3–4 50:00 at RPE 5 20:00 at RPE 2–3

	MONDAY	TUESDAY	WEDNESDAY	THURSDAY
9	Rest	**Accelerations** 5:00 at RPE 2–3 15:00 at RPE 3–4 11:00 acceleration 10:00 at RPE 2–3 6:00 acceleration 3:00 acceleration 20:00 at RPE 2–3 **Recovery Run** 25:00 at RPE 2–3	**Foundation Run** 5:00 at RPE 2–3 55:00 at RPE 3–4	**Foundation Run** 5:00 at RPE 2–3 55:00 at RPE 3–4
10	**Recovery Run** 40:00 at RPE 2–3	**The Prefontaine** 1 km at RPE 2–3 4 km at RPE 3–4 ? × 200m at RPE 9 / 200m at RPE 6 1 km at RPE 2–3 4 km at RPE 3–4 *(? = Go to failure)* **Recovery Run** 35:00 at RPE 2–3	**Foundation Run** 5:00 at RPE 2–3 55:00 at RPE 3–4	**Foundation Run** 5:00 at RPE 2–3 1:10:00 at RPE 3–4
11	**Recovery Run** 40:00 at RPE 2–3	**5K Pace Intervals** 1 km at RPE 2–3 3 km at RPE 3–4 6 × (0.8 km at 5KP / 1:00 rest) 4 km at RPE 2–3 **Recovery Run** 30:00 at RPE 2–3	**Foundation Run** 5:00 at RPE 2–3 55:00 at RPE 3–4	**Foundation Run** 5:00 at RPE 2–3 55:00 at RPE 3–4
12	Rest	**Fartleks** 5:00 at RPE 2–3 15:00 at RPE 3–4 10 × 1:00 at RPE 7–8 / 2:00 at RPE 2–3 20:00 at RPE 3–4	**Foundation Run** 5:00 at RPE 2–3 40:00 at RPE 3–4	**Fast Finish Run** 5:00 at RPE 2–3 30:00 at RPE 3–4 5:00 at RPE 6–7

FRIDAY	SATURDAY	SUNDAY

Fartleks
5:00 at RPE 2–3
15:00 at RPE 3–4
1:00 at CV, 1:00 at RPE 2–3
2:00 at LTP, 1:00 at RPE 2–3
3:00 at SSP, 1:00 at RPE 2–3
2:00 at LTP, 1:00 at RPE 2–3
1:00 at CV, 1:00 at RPE 2–3
2:00 at LTP, 1:00 at RPE 2–3
3:00 at SSP, 1:00 at RPE 2–3
20:00 at RPE 3–4

Recovery Run
25:00 at RPE 2–3

Foundation Run
5:00 at RPE 2–3
55:00 at RPE 3–4

Endurance Run
5:00 at RPE 2–3
1:30:00 at RPE 3–4
5:00 at RPE 4–5

10K Relaxed Time Trial
1 km at RPE 2–3
3 km at RPE 3–4
10 km at 95% effort
4 km at RPE 2–3

Recovery Run
35:00 at RPE 2–3

Foundation Run
5:00 at RPE 2–3
55:00 at RPE 3–4

Progression Fartleks
5:00 at RPE 2–3
15:00 at RPE 3–4
2 × (3:00 at RPE 4–5 /
   1:00 at RPE 2–3)
2 × (4:00 at RPE 5–6 /
   1:00 at RPE 2–3)
2 × (5:00 at RPE 6–7 /
   1:00 at RPE 2–3)
2 × (6:00 at RPE 7–8 /
   1:00 at RPE 2–3)
20:00 at RPE 2–3

10K Pace Intervals
1 km at RPE 2–3
3 km at RPE 3–4
10 × (1 km at 10KP / 1:00 rest)
4 km at RPE 2–3

Recovery Run
30:00 at RPE 2–3

Foundation Run
5:00 at RPE 2–3
55:00 at RPE 3–4

Endurance Run
5:00 at RPE 2–3
1:00:00 at RPE 3–4
5:00 at RPE 4–5

Foundation Run
5:00 at RPE 2–3
15:00 at RPE 3–4

10K Race

Rest

11

Half-Marathon Training Plans

The four training plans presented in this chapter are designed to help runners master the art of pacing and find their limit at the half-marathon distance. The various levels cover the needs of everyone from first-timers to elites. Refer back to Chapter 6 for details on the RPE-based intensity scale used throughout the plans and for full explanations of certain terms and workout types. Online versions of the plans are available for separate purchase on the 80/20 Endurance website. Additionally, device-compatible free versions of the individual workouts can be found at 8020endurance.com/on-pace-workouts.

Half Marathon

This plan is appropriate for beginning runners preparing for their first half-marathon event and for more experienced runners who need or prefer a relatively low-volume training program for any reason. Before starting the plan, be sure to build your training to the point where you're comfortably able to run five days a week for up to 40 minutes.

	MONDAY	TUESDAY	WEDNESDAY	THURSDAY
1	Rest	**Progression Run** 5:00 at RPE 2–3 10:00 at RPE 3–4 8:00 at SSP 4:00 at LTP 2:00 at CV 5:00 at RPE 2–3	**Foundation Run** 5:00 at RPE 2–3 25:00 at RPE 3–4	Rest
2	Rest	**Progression Run** 5:00 at RPE 2–3 20:00 at RPE 3–4 4:00 at LTP 2:00 at CV 1:00 at MAS 5:00 at RPE 2–3	**Foundation Run** 5:00 at RPE 2–3 30:00 at RPE 3–4	Rest
3	Rest	**Fartleks** 5:00 at RPE 2–3 5:00 at RPE 3–4 1:00 at CV, 1:00 at RPE 2–3 2:00 at LTP, 1:00 at RPE 2–3 3:00 at SSP, 1:00 at RPE 2–3 2:00 at LTP, 1:00 at RPE 2–3 1:00 at CV, 1:00 at RPE 2–3 10:00 at RPE 3–4	**Foundation Run** 5:00 at RPE 2–3 25:00 at RPE 3–4	Rest
4	Rest	**Critical Velocity Intervals** 5:00 at RPE 2–3 5:00 at RPE 3–4 4 × 4:00 at RPE 6–7* / 2:00 at RPE 2–3 10:00 at RPE 2–3 *Precision Splitting	**Foundation Run** 5:00 at RPE 2–3 30:00 at RPE 3–4	Rest

5	Rest	**Progression Fartleks**
		5:00 at RPE 2–3
		5:00 at RPE 3–4
		2 × (3:00 at RPE 4–5 /
		  1:00 at RPE 2–3)
		2 × (4:00 at RPE 5–6 /
		  1:00 at RPE 2–3)
		10:00 at RPE 2–3
			Foundation Run
			5:00 at RPE 2–3
			35:00 at RPE 3–4
				Rest

LEVEL

SSP Steady State Pace
LTP Lactate Threshold Pace
CV Critical Velocity
MAS Maximal Aerobic Speed

5KP 5K Pace

FRIDAY	SATURDAY	SUNDAY
Fartleks 5:00 at RPE 2–3 5:00 at RPE 3–4 6 × 0:20 at RPE 8–9 / 1:40 at RPE 2–3 10:00 at RPE 3–4	**Foundation Run** 5:00 at RPE 2–3 25:00 at RPE 3–4	**Endurance Run** 5:00 at RPE 2–3 30:00 at RPE 3–4 5:00 at RPE 4–5
Fartleks 5:00 at RPE 2–3 5:00 at RPE 3–4 6 × 1:00 at RPE 7–8 / 2:00 at RPE 2–3 10:00 at RPE 3–4	**Foundation Run** 5:00 at RPE 2–3 30:00 at RPE 3–4	**Endurance Run** 5:00 at RPE 2–3 40:00 at RPE 3–4 5:00 at RPE 4–5
Hill Repetitions 5:00 at RPE 2–3 5:00 at RPE 3–4 6 × 0:30 uphill at RPE 8–9* / 1:30 at RPE 2–3 10:00 at RPE 2–3 *Stretch Intervals*	**Foundation Run** 5:00 at RPE 2–3 25:00 at RPE 3–4	**Endurance Run** 5:00 at RPE 2–3 35:00 at RPE 3–4 5:00 at RPE 4–5
VO₂max Intervals 5:00 at RPE 2–3 5:00 at RPE 3–4 4 × 2:00 at RPE 7–8* / 2:00 at RPE 2–3 10:00 at RPE 2–3 *Precision Splitting*	**Foundation Run** 5:00 at RPE 2–3 30:00 at RPE 3–4	**Endurance Run** 5:00 at RPE 2–3 50:00 at RPE 3–4 5:00 at RPE 4–5
Accelerations 5:00 at RPE 2–3 5:00 at RPE 3–4 11:00 acceleration 10:00 at RPE 2–3 3:00 acceleration 10:00 at RPE 2–3	**Foundation Run** 5:00 at RPE 2–3 35:00 at RPE 3–4	**Endurance Run** 5:00 at RPE 2–3 1:00:00 at RPE 3–4 5:00 at RPE 4–5

	MONDAY	TUESDAY	WEDNESDAY	THURSDAY
6	Rest	**Progression Run** 5:00 at RPE 2–3 15:00 at RPE 3–4 12:00 at SSP 8:00 at LTP 4:00 at CV 5:00 at RPE 2–3	**Foundation Run** 5:00 at RPE 2–3 30:00 at RPE 3–4	Rest
7	Rest	**Tempo Run** 5:00 at RPE 2–3 5:00 at RPE 3–4 12:00 at RPE 6 5:00 at RPE 2–3 12:00 at RPE 6 10:00 at RPE 2–3	**Foundation Run** 5:00 at RPE 2–3 35:00 at RPE 3–4	Rest
8	Rest	**Steady State Run** 5:00 at RPE 2–3 5:00 at RPE 3–4 30:00 at RPE 5 10:00 at RPE 2–3	**Foundation Run** 5:00 at RPE 2–3 40:00 at RPE 3–4	Rest
9	Rest	**Fartleks** 5:00 at RPE 2–3 5:00 at RPE 3–4 1:00 at CV, 1:00 at RPE 2–3 2:00 at LTP, 1:00 at RPE 2–3 3:00 at SSP, 1:00 at RPE 2–3 2:00 at LTP, 1:00 at RPE 2–3 1:00 at CV, 1:00 at RPE 2–3 2:00 at LTP, 1:00 at RPE 2–3 1:00 at CV, 1:00 at RPE 2–3 10:00 at RPE 3–4	**Foundation Run** 5:00 at RPE 2–3 35:00 at RPE 3–4	Rest
10	Rest	**Critical Velocity Intervals** 5:00 at RPE 2–3 5:00 at RPE 3–4 5 × 4:00 at RPE 6–7* / 2:00 at RPE 2–3 10:00 at RPE 2–3 *Precision Splitting*	**Foundation Run** 5:00 at RPE 2–3 40:00 at RPE 3–4	Rest

11	Rest	**Progression Fartleks**
		5:00 at RPE 2–3
		5:00 at RPE 3–4
		2 × (3:00 at RPE 4–5 /
		  1:00 at RPE 2–3)
		2 × (4:00 at RPE 5–6 /
		  1:00 at RPE 2–3)
		2 × (5:00 at RPE 6–7 /
		  1:00 at RPE 2–3)
		10:00 at RPE 2–3
			Foundation Run
			5:00 at RPE 2–3
			40:00 at RPE 3–4
				Rest

Speed Intervals
5:00 at RPE 2–3
5:00 at RPE 3–4
6 × 0:45 at RPE 8–9* /
  1:45 at RPE 2–3
10:00 at RPE 2–3
Stretch Intervals

Foundation Run
5:00 at RPE 2–3
30:00 at RPE 3–4

Endurance Run
5:00 at RPE 2–3
50:00 at RPE 3–4
5:00 at RPE 4–5

5K Pace Intervals
1 km at RPE 2–3
1 km at RPE 3–4
8 × (0.6 km at 5KP* / 1:00 rest)
2 km at RPE 2–3
Precision Splitting

Foundation Run
5:00 at RPE 2–3
35:00 at RPE 3–4

Endurance Run
5:00 at RPE 2–3
1:10:00 at RPE 3–4
5:00 at RPE 4–5

VO₂max Intervals
5:00 at RPE 2–3
5:00 at RPE 3–4
5 × 2:00 at RPE 7–8* /
  2:00 at RPE 2–3
10:00 at RPE 2–3
Precision Splitting

Foundation Run
5:00 at RPE 2–3
40:00 at RPE 3–4

Endurance Run
5:00 at RPE 2–3
1:20:00 at RPE 3–4
5:00 at RPE 4–5

Hill Repetitions
5:00 at RPE 2–3
5:00 at RPE 3–4
6 × 1:00 uphill at RPE 8–9* /
  2:00 at RPE 2–3
10:00 at RPE 2–3
Stretch Intervals

Foundation Run
5:00 at RPE 2–3
35:00 at RPE 3–4

Endurance Run
5:00 at RPE 2–3
1:00:00 at RPE 3–4
5:00 at RPE 4–5

5K Pace Intervals
1 km at RPE 2–3
1 km at RPE 3–4
6 × (0.8 km at 5KP* / 1:00 rest)
2 km at RPE 2–3
Precision Splitting

Foundation Run
5:00 at RPE 2–3
40:00 at RPE 3–4

Endurance Run
5:00 at RPE 2–3
1:30:00 at RPE 3–4
5:00 at RPE 4–5

Accelerations
5:00 at RPE 2–3
5:00 at RPE 3–4
11:00 acceleration
10:00 at RPE 2–3
6:00 acceleration
10:00 at RPE 2–3

Foundation Run
5:00 at RPE 2–3
40:00 at RPE 3–4

Endurance Run
5:00 at RPE 2–3
1:40:00 at RPE 3–4
5:00 at RPE 4–5

Half Marathon

	MONDAY	TUESDAY	WEDNESDAY	THURSDAY
12	Rest	**Progression Run** 5:00 at RPE 2–3 30:00 at RPE 3–4 8:00 at LTP 4:00 at CV 2:00 at MAS 5:00 at RPE 2–3	**Foundation Run** 5:00 at RPE 2–3 35:00 at RPE 3–4	Rest
13	Rest	**Tempo Run** 5:00 at RPE 2–3 5:00 at RPE 3–4 14:00 at RPE 6 5:00 at RPE 2–3 14:00 at RPE 6 10:00 at RPE 2–3	**Foundation Run** 5:00 at RPE 2–3 40:00 at RPE 3–4	Rest
14	Rest	**Steady State Run** 5:00 at RPE 2–3 5:00 at RPE 3–4 40:00 at RPE 5 10:00 at RPE 2–3	**Foundation Run** 5:00 at RPE 2–3 40:00 at RPE 3–4	Rest
15	Rest	**Fartleks** 5:00 at RPE 2–3 5:00 at RPE 3–4 6 × 1:00 at RPE 7–8 / 2:00 at RPE 2–3 10:00 at RPE 3–4	**Foundation Run** 5:00 at RPE 2–3 40:00 at RPE 3–4	Rest

FRIDAY	SATURDAY	SUNDAY

Speed Intervals
5:00 at RPE 2–3
5:00 at RPE 3–4
8 × 0:45 at RPE 8–9* /
  1:45 at RPE 2–3
10:00 at RPE 2–3
Stretch Intervals

Foundation Run
5:00 at RPE 2–3
35:00 at RPE 3–4

Endurance Run
5:00 at RPE 2–3
1:10:00 at RPE 3–4
5:00 at RPE 4–5

VO₂max Intervals
5:00 at RPE 2–3
5:00 at RPE 3–4
5 × 2:00 at RPE 7–8* /
  2:00 at RPE 2–3
10:00 at RPE 2–3
Precision Splitting

Foundation Run
5:00 at RPE 2–3
40:00 at RPE 3–4

Endurance Run
5:00 at RPE 2–3
1:50:00 at RPE 3–4
5:00 at RPE 4–5

Relaxed 5K Time Trial
1 km at RPE 2–3
1 km at RPE 3–4
5 km at 95% effort
2 km at RPE 2–3

Foundation Run
5:00 at RPE 2–3
40:00 at RPE 3–4

Endurance Run
5:00 at RPE 2–3
1:10:00 at RPE 3–4
5:00 at RPE 4–5

Fast Finish Run
5:00 at RPE 2–3
10:00 at RPE 3–4
5:00 at RPE 6–7

Foundation Run
5:00 at RPE 2–3
15:00 at RPE 3–4

Half-Marathon Race

Half Marathon

Half Marathon

This plan is designed for runners who are ready to take their training load up a notch in order to improve their half-marathon time. Before starting the plan, be sure to build your training to the point where you're comfortably able to run six days a week for up to 1 hour.

	MONDAY	TUESDAY	WEDNESDAY	THURSDAY
1	Rest	**Progression Run** 5:00 at RPE 2–3 10:00 at RPE 3–4 8:00 at SSP 4:00 at LTP 2:00 at CV 5:00 at RPE 2–3	**Foundation Run** 5:00 at RPE 2–3 25:00 at RPE 3–4	**Foundation Run** 5:00 at RPE 2–3 25:00 at RPE 3–4
2	Rest	**Progression Run** 5:00 at RPE 2–3 25:00 at RPE 3–4 4:00 at LTP 2:00 at CV 1:00 at MAS 5:00 at RPE 2–3	**Foundation Run** 5:00 at RPE 2–3 30:00 at RPE 3–4	**Foundation Run** 5:00 at RPE 2–3 30:00 at RPE 3–4
3	Rest	**Fartleks** 5:00 at RPE 2–3 5:00 at RPE 3–4 1:00 at CV, 1:00 at RPE 2–3 2:00 at LTP, 1:00 at RPE 2–3 3:00 at SSP, 1:00 at RPE 2–3 2:00 at LTP, 1:00 at RPE 2–3 1:00 at CV, 1:00 at RPE 2–3 2:00 at LTP, 1:00 at RPE 2–3 3:00 at SSP, 1:00 at RPE 2–3 10:00 at RPE 3–4	**Foundation Run** 5:00 at RPE 2–3 25:00 at RPE 3–4	**Foundation Run** 5:00 at RPE 2–3 25:00 at RPE 3–4
4	Rest	**Critical Velocity Intervals** 5:00 at RPE 2–3 5:00 at RPE 3–4 5 × 4:00 at RPE 6–7* / 2:00 at RPE 2–3 10:00 at RPE 2–3 *Precision Splitting*	**Foundation Run** 5:00 at RPE 2–3 30:00 at RPE 3–4	**Foundation Run** 5:00 at RPE 2–3 30:00 at RPE 3–4

LEVEL

SSP Steady State Pace
LTP Lactate Threshold Pace
CV Critical Velocity
MAS Maximal Aerobic Speed

5KP 5K Pace
HMP Half-Marathon Pace

FRIDAY	SATURDAY	SUNDAY
Fartleks 5:00 at RPE 2–3 5:00 at RPE 3–4 6 × 0:20 at RPE 8–9 / 1:40 at RPE 2–3 10:00 at RPE 3–4	**Foundation Run** 5:00 at RPE 2–3 25:00 at RPE 3–4	**Endurance Run** 5:00 at RPE 2–3 50:00 at RPE 3–4 5:00 at RPE 4–5
Fartleks 5:00 at RPE 2–3 5:00 at RPE 3–4 6 × 1:00 at RPE 7–8 / 2:00 at RPE 2–3 10:00 at RPE 3–4	**Foundation Run** 5:00 at RPE 2–3 30:00 at RPE 3–4	**Endurance Run** 5:00 at RPE 2–3 1:00:00 at RPE 3–4 5:00 at RPE 4–5
Hill Repetitions 5:00 at RPE 2–3 5:00 at RPE 3–4 8 × 0:30 uphill at RPE 8–9* / 1:30 at RPE 2–3 10:00 at RPE 2–3 *Stretch Intervals*	**Foundation Run** 5:00 at RPE 2–3 25:00 at RPE 3–4	**Endurance Run** 5:00 at RPE 2–3 50:00 at RPE 3–4 5:00 at RPE 4–5
VO$_2$max Intervals 5:00 at RPE 2–3 5:00 at RPE 3–4 5 × 2:00 at RPE 7–8* / 2:00 at RPE 2–3 10:00 at RPE 2–3 *Precision Splitting*	**Foundation Run** 5:00 at RPE 2–3 30:00 at RPE 3–4	**Endurance Run** 5:00 at RPE 2–3 1:10:00 at RPE 3–4 5:00 at RPE 4–5

	MONDAY	TUESDAY	WEDNESDAY	THURSDAY

5	Rest	**Progression Fartleks**
		5:00 at RPE 2–3
		5:00 at RPE 3–4
		2 × (3:00 at RPE 4–5 /
		  1:00 at RPE 2–3)
		2 × (4:00 at RPE 5–6 /
		  1:00 at RPE 2–3)
		10:00 at RPE 2–3
			Foundation Run
			5:00 at RPE 2–3
			35:00 at RPE 3–4
				Foundation Run
				5:00 at RPE 2–3
				35:00 at RPE 3–4

6	Rest	**Progression Run** 5:00 at RPE 2–3 20:00 at RPE 3–4 12:00 at SSP 8:00 at LTP 4:00 at CV 5:00 at RPE 2–3	**Foundation Run** 5:00 at RPE 2–3 30:00 at RPE 3–4	**Foundation Run** 5:00 at RPE 2–3 30:00 at RPE 3–4
7	Rest	**Tempo Run** 5:00 at RPE 2–3 5:00 at RPE 3–4 14:00 at RPE 6 5:00 at RPE 2–3 14:00 at RPE 6 10:00 at RPE 2–3	**Foundation Run** 5:00 at RPE 2–3 35:00 at RPE 3–4	**Foundation Run** 5:00 at RPE 2–3 35:00 at RPE 3–4
8	Rest	**Steady State Run** 5:00 at RPE 2–3 5:00 at RPE 3–4 35:00 at RPE 5 10:00 at RPE 2–3	**Foundation Run** 5:00 at RPE 2–3 40:00 at RPE 3–4	**Foundation Run** 5:00 at RPE 2–3 40:00 at RPE 3–4
9	Rest	**Fartleks** 5:00 at RPE 2–3 5:00 at RPE 3–4 1:00 at CV, 1:00 at RPE 2–3 2:00 at LTP, 1:00 at RPE 2–3 3:00 at SSP, 1:00 at RPE 2–3 2:00 at LTP, 1:00 at RPE 2–3 1:00 at CV, 1:00 at RPE 2–3 2:00 at LTP, 1:00 at RPE 2–3 1:00 at CV, 1:00 at RPE 2–3 10:00 at RPE 3–4	**Foundation Run** 5:00 at RPE 2–3 35:00 at RPE 3–4	**Foundation Run** 5:00 at RPE 2–3 35:00 at RPE 3–4
10	Rest	**Critical Velocity Intervals** 5:00 at RPE 2–3 5:00 at RPE 3–4 6 × 4:00 at RPE 6–7* / 2:00 at RPE 2–3 10:00 at RPE 2–3 *Precision Splitting*	**Foundation Run** 5:00 at RPE 2–3 40:00 at RPE 3–4	**Foundation Run** 5:00 at RPE 2–3 40:00 at RPE 3–4

FRIDAY	SATURDAY	SUNDAY
Accelerations 5:00 at RPE 2–3 5:00 at RPE 3–4 11:00 acceleration 10:00 at RPE 2–3 6:00 acceleration 10:00 at RPE 2–3	**Foundation Run** 5:00 at RPE 2–3 35:00 at RPE 3–4	**Endurance Run** 5:00 at RPE 2–3 1:20:00 at RPE 3–4 5:00 at RPE 4–5
Speed Intervals 5:00 at RPE 2–3 5:00 at RPE 3–4 8 × 0:45 at RPE 8–9* / 1:45 at RPE 2–3 10:00 at RPE 2–3 *Stretch Intervals*	**Foundation Run** 5:00 at RPE 2–3 30:00 at RPE 3–4	**Endurance Run** 5:00 at RPE 2–3 1:00:00 at RPE 3–4 5:00 at RPE 4–5
5K Pace Intervals 1 km at RPE 2–3 1 km at RPE 3–4 6 × (0.8 km at 5KP* / 1:00 rest) 2 km at RPE 2–3 *Precision Splitting*	**Foundation Run** 5:00 at RPE 2–3 35:00 at RPE 3–4	**Endurance Run** 5:00 at RPE 2–3 1:30:00 at RPE 3–4 5:00 at RPE 4–5
VO₂max Intervals 5:00 at RPE 2–3 5:00 at RPE 3–4 6 × 2:00 at RPE 7–8* / 2:00 at RPE 2–3 10:00 at RPE 2–3 *Precision Splitting*	**Foundation Run** 5:00 at RPE 2–3 40:00 at RPE 3–4	**Half-Marathon Pace Run** 1 km at RPE 2–3 1 km at RPE 3–4 3 × (3 km at HMP / 1:00 rest) 2 km at RPE 2–3
Hill Repetitions 5:00 at RPE 2–3 5:00 at RPE 3–4 8 × 1:00 uphill at RPE 8–9* / 2:00 at RPE 2–3 10:00 at RPE 2–3 *Stretch Intervals*	**Foundation Run** 5:00 at RPE 2–3 35:00 at RPE 3–4	**Endurance Run** 5:00 at RPE 2–3 1:10:00 at RPE 3–4 5:00 at RPE 4–5
The Prefontaine 1 km at RPE 2–3 1 km at RPE 3–4 ? × 200m at RPE 9 / 200m at RPE 6 1 km at RPE 2–3 1 km at RPE 3–4 (? = Go to failure)	**Foundation Run** 5:00 at RPE 2–3 40:00 at RPE 3–4	**Endurance Run** 5:00 at RPE 2–3 1:40:00 at RPE 3–4 5:00 at RPE 4–5

Half Marathon

1

	MONDAY	TUESDAY	WEDNESDAY	THURSDAY

11	Rest	**Progression Fartleks**
		5:00 at RPE 2–3
		5:00 at RPE 3–4
		2 × (3:00 at RPE 4–5 /
		  1:00 at RPE 2–3)
		2 × (4:00 at RPE 5–6 /
		  1:00 at RPE 2–3)
		2 × (5:00 at RPE 6–7 /
		  1:00 at RPE 2–3)
		10:00 at RPE 2–3
			Foundation Run
			5:00 at RPE 2–3
			45:00 at RPE 3–4
				Foundation Run
				5:00 at RPE 2–3
				45:00 at RPE 3–4

12	Rest	**Progression Run** 5:00 at RPE 2–3 30:00 at RPE 3–4 8:00 at LTP 4:00 at CV 2:00 at MAS 5:00 at RPE 2–3	**Foundation Run** 5:00 at RPE 2–3 40:00 at RPE 3–4	**Foundation Run** 5:00 at RPE 2–3 40:00 at RPE 3–4
13	Rest	**Tempo Run** 5:00 at RPE 2–3 5:00 at RPE 3–4 16:00 at RPE 6 5:00 at RPE 2–3 16:00 at RPE 6 10:00 at RPE 2–3	**Foundation Run** 5:00 at RPE 2–3 45:00 at RPE 3–4	**Foundation Run** 5:00 at RPE 2–3 45:00 at RPE 3–4
14	Rest	**Steady State Run** 5:00 at RPE 2–3 5:00 at RPE 3–4 45:00 at RPE 5 10:00 at RPE 2–3	**Foundation Run** 5:00 at RPE 2–3 40:00 at RPE 3–4	**Foundation Run** 5:00 at RPE 2–3 40:00 at RPE 3–4
15	Rest	**Fartleks** 5:00 at RPE 2–3 5:00 at RPE 3–4 8 × 1:00 at RPE 7–8 / 2:00 at RPE 2–3 10:00 at RPE 3–4	**Foundation Run** 5:00 at RPE 2–3 35:00 at RPE 3–4	**Foundation Run** 5:00 at RPE 2–3 25:00 at RPE 3–4

FRIDAY	SATURDAY	SUNDAY
Speed Intervals 5:00 at RPE 2–3 5:00 at RPE 3–4 8 × 0:45 at RPE 8–9* / 1:45 at RPE 2–3 10:00 at RPE 2–3 *Stretch Intervals*	**Foundation Run** 5:00 at RPE 2–3 45:00 at RPE 3–4	**Endurance Run** 5:00 at RPE 2–3 1:50:00 at RPE 3–4 5:00 at RPE 4–5
Accelerations 5:00 at RPE 2–3 5:00 at RPE 3–4 11:00 acceleration 10:00 at RPE 2–3 6:00 acceleration 10:00 at RPE 2–3	**Foundation Run** 5:00 at RPE 2–3 40:00 at RPE 3–4	**Endurance Run** 5:00 at RPE 2–3 1:10:00 at RPE 3–4 5:00 at RPE 4–5
VO₂max Intervals 5:00 at RPE 2–3 5:00 at RPE 3–4 6 × 2:00 at RPE 7–8* / 2:00 at RPE 2–3 10:00 at RPE 2–3 *Precision Splitting*	**Foundation Run** 5:00 at RPE 2–3 45:00 at RPE 3–4	**Half-Marathon Pace Run** 1 km at RPE 2–3 1 km at RPE 3–4 2 × (5 km at HMP / 1:00 rest) 2 km at RPE 2–3
Relaxed 5K Time Trial 1 km at RPE 2–3 1 km at RPE 3–4 5 km at 95% effort 2 km at RPE 2–3	**Foundation Run** 5:00 at RPE 2–3 40:00 at RPE 3–4	**Endurance Run** 5:00 at RPE 2–3 1:10:00 at RPE 3–4 5:00 at RPE 4–5
Fast Finish Run 5:00 at RPE 2–3 15:00 at RPE 3–4 5:00 at RPE 6–7	**Foundation Run** 5:00 at RPE 2–3 15:00 at RPE 3–4	**Half-Marathon Race**

Half Marathon

This plan is a good fit for experienced competitive runners who are prepared to train hard in pursuit of improved half-marathon performance. Before starting the plan, be sure to build your training to the point where you're comfortably able to run seven days a week for up to 80 minutes.

	MONDAY	TUESDAY	WEDNESDAY	THURSDAY
1	**Recovery Run** 30:00 at RPE 2–3	**Progression Run** 5:00 at RPE 2–3 25:00 at RPE 3–4 8:00 at SSP 4:00 at LTP 2:00 at CV 5:00 at RPE 2–3	**Foundation Run** 5:00 at RPE 2–3 40:00 at RPE 3–4	**Foundation Run** 5:00 at RPE 2–3 40:00 at RPE 3–4
2	**Recovery Run** 30:00 at RPE 2–3	**Progression Run** 5:00 at RPE 2–3 35:00 at RPE 3–4 4:00 at LTP 2:00 at CV 1:00 at MAS 5:00 at RPE 2–3	**Foundation Run** 5:00 at RPE 2–3 45:00 at RPE 3–4	**Foundation Run** 5:00 at RPE 2–3 45:00 at RPE 3–4
3	Rest	**Fartleks** 5:00 at RPE 2–3 10:00 at RPE 3–4 1:00 at CV, 1:00 at RPE 2–3 2:00 at LTP, 1:00 at RPE 2–3 3:00 at SSP, 1:00 at RPE 2–3 2:00 at LTP, 1:00 at RPE 2–3 1:00 at CV, 1:00 at RPE 2–3 2:00 at LTP, 1:00 at RPE 2–3 3:00 at SSP, 1:00 at RPE 2–3 15:00 at RPE 3–4	**Foundation Run** 5:00 at RPE 2–3 40:00 at RPE 3–4	**Foundation Run** 5:00 at RPE 2–3 40:00 at RPE 3–4
4	**Recovery Run** 30:00 at RPE 2–3	**Critical Velocity Intervals** 5:00 at RPE 2–3 10:00 at RPE 3–4 6 × 4:00* at RPE 6–7 / 2:00 at RPE 2–3 15:00 at RPE 2–3 *Precision Splitting*	**Foundation Run** 5:00 at RPE 2–3 45:00 at RPE 3–4	**Foundation Run** 5:00 at RPE 2–3 45:00 at RPE 3–4

LEVEL

SSP   Steady State Pace
LTP   Lactate Threshold Pace
CV   Critical Velocity
MAS   Maximal Aerobic Speed

5KP   5K Pace
HMP   Half-Marathon Pace

FRIDAY	SATURDAY	SUNDAY
Fartleks 5:00 at RPE 2–3 10:00 at RPE 3–4 8 × 0:20 at RPE 8–9 / 1:40 at RPE 2–3 15:00 at RPE 3–4	**Foundation Run** 5:00 at RPE 2–3 40:00 at RPE 3–4	**Endurance Run** 5:00 at RPE 2–3 1:10:00 at RPE 3–4 5:00 at RPE 4–5
Fartleks 5:00 at RPE 2–3 10:00 at RPE 3–4 8 × 1:00 at RPE 7–8 / 2:00 at RPE 2–3 15:00 at RPE 3–4	**Foundation Run** 5:00 at RPE 2–3 45:00 at RPE 3–4	**Endurance Run** 5:00 at RPE 2–3 1:20:00 at RPE 3–4 5:00 at RPE 4–5
Hill Repetitions 5:00 at RPE 2–3 10:00 at RPE 3–4 10 × 0:30 uphill at RPE 8–9 / 1:30 at RPE 2–3 15:00 at RPE 2–3	**Foundation Run** 5:00 at RPE 2–3 40:00 at RPE 3–4	**Endurance Run** 5:00 at RPE 2–3 1:10:00 at RPE 3–4 5:00 at RPE 4–5
VO$_2$max Intervals 5:00 at RPE 2–3 10:00 at RPE 3–4 6 × 2:00* at RPE 7–8 / 2:00 at RPE 2–3 15:00 at RPE 2–3 *Precision Splitting	**Foundation Run** 5:00 at RPE 2–3 45:00 at RPE 3–4	**Endurance Run** 5:00 at RPE 2–3 1:30:00 at RPE 3–4 5:00 at RPE 4–5

Half Marathon

2

	MONDAY	TUESDAY	WEDNESDAY	THURSDAY
5	**Recovery Run** 30:00 at RPE 2–3	**Progression Fartleks** 5:00 at RPE 2–3 10:00 at RPE 3–4 2 × (3:00 at RPE 4–5 / 1:00 at RPE 2–3) 2 × (4:00 at RPE 5–6 / 1:00 at RPE 2–3) 2 × (5:00 at RPE 5–6 / 1:00 at RPE 2–3) 15:00 at RPE 2–3	**Foundation Run** 5:00 at RPE 2–3 50:00 at RPE 3–4	**Foundation Run** 5:00 at RPE 2–3 50:00 at RPE 3–4
6	Rest	**Progression Run** 5:00 at RPE 2–3 25:00 at RPE 3–4 12:00 at SSP 8:00 at LTP 4:00 at CV 5:00 at RPE 2–3	**Foundation Run** 5:00 at RPE 2–3 45:00 at RPE 3–4	**Foundation Run** 5:00 at RPE 2–3 45:00 at RPE 3–4
7	**Recovery Run** 30:00 at RPE 2–3	**Tempo Run** 5:00 at RPE 2–3 10:00 at RPE 3–4 16:00 at RPE 6 5:00 at RPE 2–3 16:00 at RPE 6 15:00 at RPE 2–3	**Foundation Run** 5:00 at RPE 2–3 50:00 at RPE 3–4	**Foundation Run** 5:00 at RPE 2–3 50:00 at RPE 3–4
8	**Recovery Run** 30:00 at RPE 2–3	**Steady State Run** 5:00 at RPE 2–3 10:00 at RPE 3–4 40:00 at RPE 5 15:00 at RPE 2–3	**Foundation Run** 5:00 at RPE 2–3 55:00 at RPE 3–4	**Foundation Run** 5:00 at RPE 2–3 55:00 at RPE 3–4
9	Rest	**Fartleks** 5:00 at RPE 2–3 10:00 at RPE 3–4 1:00 at CV, 1:00 at RPE 2–3 2:00 at LTP, 1:00 at RPE 2–3 3:00 at SSP, 1:00 at RPE 2–3 2:00 at LTP, 1:00 at RPE 2–3 1:00 at CV, 1:00 at RPE 2–3 2:00 at LTP, 1:00 at RPE 2–3 1:00 at CV, s1:00 at RPE 2–3 15:00 at RPE 3–4	**Foundation Run** 5:00 at RPE 2–3 45:00 at RPE 3–4	**Foundation Run** 5:00 at RPE 2–3 45:00 at RPE 3–4
10	**Recovery Run** 30:00 at RPE 2–3	**Critical Velocity Intervals** 5:00 at RPE 2–3 10:00 at RPE 3–4 7 × 4:00* at RPE 6–7 / 2:00 at RPE 2–3 15:00 at RPE 2–3 *Precision Splitting*	**Foundation Run** 5:00 at RPE 2–3 55:00 at RPE 3–4	**Foundation Run** 5:00 at RPE 2–3 55:00 at RPE 3–4

FRIDAY	SATURDAY	SUNDAY
Accelerations 5:00 at RPE 2–3 10:00 at RPE 3–4 11:00 acceleration 10:00 at RPE 2–3 6:00 acceleration 15:00 at RPE 2–3	**Foundation Run** 5:00 at RPE 2–3 50:00 at RPE 3–4	**Endurance Run** 5:00 at RPE 2–3 1:40:00 at RPE 3–4 5:00 at RPE 4–5
Speed Intervals 5:00 at RPE 2–3 10:00 at RPE 3–4 8 × 1:00* at RPE 8–9 / 2:00 at RPE 2–3 15:00 at RPE 2–3 *Stretch Intervals*	**Foundation Run** 5:00 at RPE 2–3 45:00 at RPE 3–4	**Endurance Run** 5:00 at RPE 2–3 1:20:00 at RPE 3–4 5:00 at RPE 4–5
5K Pace Intervals 1 km at RPE 2–3 2.5 km at RPE 3–4 6 × (0.8 km at 5KP* / 1:00 rest) 3.5 km at RPE 2–3 *Precision Splitting*	**Foundation Run** 5:00 at RPE 2–3 50:00 at RPE 3–4	**Half-Marathon Pace Run** 1 km at RPE 2–3 2.5 km at RPE 3–4 3 × (3 km at HMP / 1:00 rest) 3.5 km at RPE 2–3
VO₂max Intervals 5:00 at RPE 2–3 10:00 at RPE 3–4 7 × 2:00* at RPE 7–8 / 2:00 at RPE 2–3 15:00 at RPE 2–3 *Precision Splitting*	**Foundation Run** 5:00 at RPE 2–3 55:00 at RPE 3–4	**Endurance Run** 5:00 at RPE 2–3 1:50:00 at RPE 3–4 5:00 at RPE 4–5
Hill Repetitions 5:00 at RPE 2–3 10:00 at RPE 3–4 10 × 1:00 uphill at RPE 8–9* / 2:00 at RPE 2–3 15:00 at RPE 2–3 *Stretch Intervals*	**Foundation Run** 5:00 at RPE 2–3 45:00 at RPE 3–4	**Depletion Run** 5:00 at RPE 2–3 1:10:00 at RPE 3–4 5:00 at RPE 4–5 *No calories before or during*
The Prefontaine 1 km at RPE 2–3 2.5 km at RPE 3–4 ? × 200m at RPE 9 / 200m at RPE 6 1 km at RPE 2–3 2.5 km at RPE 3–4 *(? = Go to failure)*	**Foundation Run** 5:00 at RPE 2–3 55:00 at RPE 3–4	**Half-Marathon Pace Run** 1 km at RPE 2–3 2.5 km at RPE 3–4 2 × (5 km at HMP / 1:00 rest) 3.5 km at RPE 2–3

Half Marathon

2

	MONDAY	TUESDAY	WEDNESDAY	THURSDAY
11	**Recovery Run** 30:00 at RPE 2–3	**Tempo Run** 5:00 at RPE 2–3 10:00 at RPE 3–4 20:00 at RPE 6 5:00 at RPE 2–3 20:00 at RPE 6 15:00 at RPE 2–3	**Foundation Run** 5:00 at RPE 2–3 55:00 at RPE 3–4	**Foundation Run** 5:00 at RPE 2–3 55:00 at RPE 3–4

12	Rest	**Progression Fartleks**
		5:00 at RPE 2–3
		10:00 at RPE 3–4
		2 × (3:00 at RPE 4–5 /
		  1:00 at RPE 2–3)
		2 × (4:00 at RPE 5–6 /
		  1:00 at RPE 2–3)
		2 × (5:00 at RPE 6–7 /
		  1:00 at RPE 2–3)
		15:00 at RPE 2–3
			Foundation Run
			5:00 at RPE 2–3
			50:00 at RPE 3–4
				Foundation Run
				5:00 at RPE 2–3
				50:00 at RPE 3–4

13	**Recovery Run** 30:00 at RPE 2–3	**Relaxed 10K Time Trial** 1 km at RPE 2–3 2.5 km at RPE 3–4 10 km at 95% effort 3.5 km at RPE 2–3	**Foundation Run** 5:00 at RPE 2–3 55:00 at RPE 3–4	**Foundation Run** 5:00 at RPE 2–3 55:00 at RPE 3–4
14	**Recovery Run** 30:00 at RPE 2–3	**Steady State Run** 5:00 at RPE 2–3 10:00 at RPE 3–4 50:00 at RPE 5 15:00 at RPE 2–3	**Foundation Run** 5:00 at RPE 2–3 55:00 at RPE 3–4	**Foundation Run** 5:00 at RPE 2–3 50:00 at RPE 3–4
15	Rest	**Fartleks** 5:00 at RPE 2–3 10:00 at RPE 3–4 8 × 1:00 at RPE 7–8 / 2:00 at RPE 2–3 15:00 at RPE 3–4	**Foundation Run** 5:00 at RPE 2–3 40:00 at RPE 3–4	**Foundation Run** 5:00 at RPE 2–3 40:00 at RPE 3–4

FRIDAY	SATURDAY	SUNDAY
Accelerations 5:00 at RPE 2–3 10:00 at RPE 3–4 11:00 acceleration 10:00 at RPE 2–3 6:00 acceleration 10:00 at RPE 2–3 3:00 acceleration 15:00 at RPE 2–3	**Foundation Run** 5:00 at RPE 2–3 55:00 at RPE 3–4	**Endurance Run** 5:00 at RPE 2–3 2:05:00 at RPE 3–4 5:00 at RPE 4–5
Speed Intervals 5:00 at RPE 2–3 5:00 at RPE 3–4 12 × 0:45 at RPE 8–9* / 1:45 at RPE 2–3 10:00 at RPE 2–3 *Stretch Intervals*	**Foundation Run** 5:00 at RPE 2–3 50:00 at RPE 3–4	**Depletion Run** 5:00 at RPE 2–3 1:30:00 at RPE 3–4 5:00 at RPE 4–5 *No calories before or during*
VO₂max Intervals 5:00 at RPE 2–3 10:00 at RPE 3–4 6 × 2:00 at RPE 7–8* / 2:00 at RPE 2–3 15:00 at RPE 2–3 *Precision Splitting*	**Foundation Run** 5:00 at RPE 2–3 55:00 at RPE 3–4	**Half-Marathon Pace Run** 1 km at RPE 2–3 2.5 km at RPE 3–4 13 km at HMP 3.5 km at RPE 2–3
Relaxed 5K Time Trial 1 km at RPE 2–3 1 km at RPE 3–4 5 km at 95% effort 2 km at RPE 2–3	**Foundation Run** 5:00 at RPE 2–3 45:00 at RPE 3–4	**Endurance Run** 5:00 at RPE 2–3 1:10:00 at RPE 3–4 5:00 at RPE 4–5
Fast Finish Run 5:00 at RPE 2–3 20:00 at RPE 3–4 10:00 at RPE 6	**Foundation Run** 5:00 at RPE 2–3 15:00 at RPE 3–4	**Half-Marathon Race**

Half Marathon

This plan was designed for serious competitive runners seeking the absolute limit of their potential at the half-marathon distance. Before starting the plan, be sure to build your training to the point where you're comfortably able to run nine times per week for up to 80 minutes.

	MONDAY	TUESDAY	WEDNESDAY	THURSDAY
1	**Recovery Run** 40:00 at RPE 2–3	**Progression Run** 5:00 at RPE 2–3 35:00 at RPE 3–4 8:00 at SSP 4:00 at LTP 2:00 at CV 5:00 at RPE 2–3 **Recovery Run** 20:00 at RPE 2–3	**Foundation Run** 5:00 at RPE 2–3 55:00 at RPE 3–4	**Foundation Run** 5:00 at RPE 2–3 55:00 at RPE 3–4
2	**Recovery Run** 40:00 at RPE 2–3	**Progression Run** 5:00 at RPE 2–3 35:00 at RPE 3–4 4:00 at LTP 2:00 at CV 1:00 at MAS 5:00 at RPE 2–3 **Recovery Run** 20:00 at RPE 2–3	**Foundation Run** 5:00 at RPE 2–3 55:00 at RPE 3–4	**Foundation Run** 5:00 at RPE 2–3 55:00 at RPE 3–4
3	Rest	**Fartleks** 5:00 at RPE 2–3 15:00 at RPE 3–4 1:00 at CV, 1:00 at RPE 2–3 2:00 at LTP, 1:00 at RPE 2–3 3:00 at SSP, 1:00 at RPE 2–3 2:00 at LTP, 1:00 at RPE 2–3 1:00 at CV, 1:00 at RPE 2–3 2:00 at LTP, 1:00 at RPE 2–3 3:00 at SSP, 1:00 at RPE 2–3 20:00 at RPE 3–4 **Recovery Run** 20:00 at RPE 2–3	**Foundation Run** 5:00 at RPE 2–3 45:00 at RPE 3–4	**Foundation Run** 5:00 at RPE 2–3 45:00 at RPE 3–4

LEVEL

SSP Steady State Pace
LTP Lactate Threshold Pace
CV Critical Velocity
MAS Maximal Aerobic Speed

5KP 5K Pace
HMP Half-Marathon Pace
MP Marathon Pace

FRIDAY	SATURDAY	SUNDAY
Fartleks 5:00 at RPE 2–3 15:00 at RPE 3–4 10 × 0:20 at RPE 8–9 / 1:40 at RPE 2–3 20:00 at RPE 3–4 **Recovery Run** 20:00 at RPE 2–3	**Foundation Run** 5:00 at RPE 2–3 55:00 at RPE 3–4	**Endurance Run** 5:00 at RPE 2–3 1:10:00 at RPE 3–4 5:00 at RPE 4–5
Fartleks 5:00 at RPE 2–3 10:00 at RPE 3–4 8 × 1:00 at RPE 7–8 / 2:00 at RPE 2–3 15:00 at RPE 3–4 **Recovery Run** 20:00 at RPE 2–3	**Foundation Run** 5:00 at RPE 2–3 55:00 at RPE 3–4	**Endurance Run** 5:00 at RPE 2–3 1:30:00 at RPE 3–4 5:00 at RPE 4–5
Hill Repetitions 5:00 at RPE 2–3 15:00 at RPE 3–4 12 × 0:30 uphill at RPE 8–9 / 1:30 at RPE 2–3 20:00 at RPE 2–3 **Recovery Run** 20:00 at RPE 2–3	**Foundation Run** 5:00 at RPE 2–3 45:00 at RPE 3–4	**Endurance Run** 5:00 at RPE 2–3 1:20:00 at RPE 3–4 5:00 at RPE 4–5

Half Marathon

3

	MONDAY	TUESDAY	WEDNESDAY	THURSDAY
4	**Recovery Run** 40:00 at RPE 2–3	**Critical Velocity Intervals** 5:00 at RPE 2–3 15:00 at RPE 3–4 7 × 4:00* at RPE 6–7 / 2:00 at RPE 2–3 20:00 at RPE 2–3 *Precision Splitting **Recovery Run** 25:00 at RPE 2–3	**Foundation Run** 5:00 at RPE 2–3 55:00 at RPE 3–4	**Foundation Run** 5:00 at RPE 2–3 1:00:00 at RPE 3–4
5	**Recovery Run** 40:00 at RPE 2–3	**Progression Fartleks** 5:00 at RPE 2–3 15:00 at RPE 3–4 2 × (3:00 at RPE 4–5 / 1:00 at RPE 2–3) 2 × (4:00 at RPE 5–6 / 1:00 at RPE 2–3) 2 × (5:00 at RPE 6–7 / 1:00 at RPE 2–3) 20:00 at RPE 2–3 **Recovery Run** 25:00 at RPE 2–3	**Foundation Run** 5:00 at RPE 2–3 55:00 at RPE 3–4	**Foundation Run** 5:00 at RPE 2–3 1:00:00 at RPE 3–4
6	Rest	**Progression Run** 5:00 at RPE 2–3 30:00 at RPE 3–4 12:00 at SSP 8:00 at LTP 4:00 at CV 5:00 at RPE 2–3 **Recovery Run** 20:00 at RPE 2–3	**Foundation Run** 5:00 at RPE 2–3 50:00 at RPE 3–4	**Foundation Run** 5:00 at RPE 2–3 50:00 at RPE 3–4
7	**Recovery Run** 40:00 at RPE 2–3	**Tempo Run** 5:00 at RPE 2–3 15:00 at RPE 3–4 18:00 at RPE 6 5:00 at RPE 2–3 18:00 at RPE 6 20:00 at RPE 2–3 **Recovery Run** 30:00 at RPE 2–3	**Foundation Run** 5:00 at RPE 2–3 55:00 at RPE 3–4	**Foundation Run** 5:00 at RPE 2–3 1:05:00 at RPE 3–4
8	**Recovery Run** 40:00 at RPE 2–3	**Steady State Run** 5:00 at RPE 2–3 15:00 at RPE 3–4 45:00 at RPE 5 20:00 at RPE 2–3 **Recovery Run** 30:00 at RPE 2–3	**Foundation Run** 5:00 at RPE 2–3 55:00 at RPE 3–4	**Foundation Run** 5:00 at RPE 2–3 1:05:00 at RPE 3–4

FRIDAY	SATURDAY	SUNDAY

FRIDAY

VO₂max Intervals
5:00 at RPE 2–3
15:00 at RPE 3–4
7 × 2:00* at RPE 7–8 /
  2:00 at RPE 2–3
20:00 at RPE 2–3
Precision Splitting

Recovery Run
25:00 at RPE 2–3

Accelerations
5:00 at RPE 2–3
15:00 at RPE 3–4
11:00 acceleration
10:00 at RPE 2–3
6:00 acceleration
10:00 at RPE 2–3
11:00 acceleration
20:00 at RPE 2–3

Recovery Run
25:00 at RPE 2–3

Speed Intervals
5:00 at RPE 2–3
15:00 at RPE 3–4
10 × 1:00* at RPE 8–9 /
  2:00 at RPE 2–3
20:00 at RPE 2–3
Stretch Intervals

Recovery Run
20:00 at RPE 2–3

5K Pace Intervals
1 km at RPE 2–3
4 km at RPE 3–4
6 × (0.8 km at 5KP* / 1:00 rest)
5 km at RPE 2–3
Precision Splitting

Recovery Run
30:00 at RPE 2–3

VO₂max Intervals
5:00 at RPE 2–3
15:00 at RPE 3–4
8 × 2:00* at RPE 7–8 /
  2:00 at RPE 2–3
20:00 at RPE 2–3
Precision Splitting

Recovery Run
30:00 at RPE 2–3

SATURDAY

Foundation Run
5:00 at RPE 2–3
55:00 at RPE 3–4

Foundation Run
5:00 at RPE 2–3
55:00 at RPE 3–4

Foundation Run
5:00 at RPE 2–3
50:00 at RPE 3–4

Foundation Run
5:00 at RPE 2–3
55:00 at RPE 3–4

Foundation Run
5:00 at RPE 2–3
55:00 at RPE 3–4

SUNDAY

Endurance Run
5:00 at RPE 2–3
1:50:00 at RPE 3–4
5:00 at RPE 4–5

Marathon Pace Run
1 km (0.6 mile) at RPE 2–3
2 km (1.2 miles) at RPE 3–4
5 × 1.5 km (0.9 mile) at MP /
  1.5 km (0.9 mile) at RPE 3–4
2 km (1.2 miles) at RPE 2–3

Depletion Run
5:00 at RPE 2–3
1:15:00 at RPE 3–4
No calories before or during

Half-Marathon Pace Run
1 km at RPE 2–3
4 km at RPE 3–4
3 × (3 km at HMP / 1:00 rest)
5 km at RPE 2–3

Endurance Run
5:00 at RPE 2–3
2:05:00 at RPE 3–4
5:00 at RPE 4–5

	MONDAY	TUESDAY	WEDNESDAY	THURSDAY
9	Rest	**Fartleks** 5:00 at RPE 2–3 15:00 at RPE 3–4 1:00 at CV, 1:00 at RPE 2–3 2:00 at LTP, 1:00 at RPE 2–3 3:00 at SSP, 1:00 at RPE 2–3 2:00 at LTP, 1:00 at RPE 2–3 1:00 at CV, 1:00 at RPE 2–3 2:00 at LTP, 1:00 at RPE 2–3 3:00 at SSP, 1:00 at RPE 2–3 2:00 at LTP, 1:00 at RPE 2–3 1:00 at CV, 1:00 at RPE 2–3 20:00 at RPE 3–4 **Recovery Run** 25:00 at RPE 2–3	**Foundation Run** 5:00 at RPE 2–3 55:00 at RPE 3–4	**Foundation Run** 5:00 at RPE 2–3 55:00 at RPE 3–4
10	**Recovery Run** 40:00 at RPE 2–3	**Critical Velocity Intervals** 5:00 at RPE 2–3 15:00 at RPE 3–4 8 × 4:00* at RPE 6–7 / 2:00 at RPE 2–3 20:00 at RPE 2–3 *Precision Splitting* **Recovery Run** 35:00 at RPE 2–3	**Foundation Run** 5:00 at RPE 2–3 55:00 at RPE 3–4	**Foundation Run** 5:00 at RPE 2–3 1:10:00 at RPE 3–4
11	**Recovery Run** 40:00 at RPE 2–3	**Tempo Run** 5:00 at RPE 2–3 15:00 at RPE 3–4 22:00 at RPE 6 5:00 at RPE 2–3 22:00 at RPE 6 20:00 at RPE 2–3 **Recovery Run** 35:00 at RPE 2–3	**Foundation Run** 5:00 at RPE 2–3 55:00 at RPE 3–4	**Foundation Run** 5:00 at RPE 2–3 1:10:00 at RPE 3–4

12	Rest	**Progression Fartleks**
		5:00 at RPE 2–3
		15:00 at RPE 3–4
		2 × (3:00 at RPE 4–5 /
		  1:00 at RPE 2–3)
		2 × (4:00 at RPE 5–6 /
		  1:00 at RPE 2–3)
		2 × (5:00 at RPE 6–7 /
		  1:00 at RPE 2–3)
		2 × (6:00 at RPE 6–7 /
		  1:00 at RPE 2–3)
		20:00 at RPE 2–3
		
		Recovery Run
		30:00 at RPE 2–3
			Foundation Run
			5:00 at RPE 2–3
			55:00 at RPE 3–4
				Foundation Run
				5:00 at RPE 2–3
				1:00:00 at RPE 3–4

FRIDAY	SATURDAY	SUNDAY

Hill Repetitions
5:00 at RPE 2–3
15:00 at RPE 3–4
10 × 1:00 uphill at RPE 8–9* /
   2:00 at RPE 2–3
20:00 at RPE 2–3
*Stretch Intervals

Recovery Run
25:00 at RPE 2–3

Foundation Run
5:00 at RPE 2–3
55:00 at RPE 3–4

Depletion Run
5:00 at RPE 2–3
1:35:00 at RPE 3–4
No calories before or during

The Prefontaine
1 km at RPE 2–3
4 km at RPE 3–4
? × 200m at RPE 9 /
   200m at RPE 6
1 km at RPE 2–3
4 km at RPE 3–4
(? = Go to failure)

Recovery Run
35:00 at RPE 2–3

Foundation Run
5:00 at RPE 2–3
55:00 at RPE 3–4

Half-Marathon Pace Run
1 km at RPE 2–3
4 km at RPE 3–4
2 × (5 km at HMP / 1:00 rest)
5 km at RPE 2–3

Accelerations
5:00 at RPE 2–3
15:00 at RPE 3–4
11:00 acceleration
10:00 at RPE 2–3
6:00 acceleration
10:00 at RPE 2–3
3:00 acceleration
20:00 at RPE 2–3

Recovery Run
35:00 at RPE 2–3

Foundation Run
5:00 at RPE 2–3
55:00 at RPE 3–4

Endurance Run
5:00 at RPE 2–3
2:25:00 at RPE 3–4
5:00 at RPE 4–5

Speed Intervals
5:00 at RPE 2–3
15:00 at RPE 3–4
12 × 0:45 at RPE 8–9* /
   1:45 at RPE 2–3
20:00 at RPE 2–3
*Stretch Intervals

Recovery Run
30:00 at RPE 2–3

Foundation Run
5:00 at RPE 2–3
55:00 at RPE 3–4

Depletion Run
5:00 at RPE 2–3
1:55:00 at RPE 3–4
No calories before or during

Half Marathon

3

	MONDAY	TUESDAY	WEDNESDAY	THURSDAY
13	**Recovery Run** 40:00 at RPE 2–3	**Relaxed 10K Time Trial** 1 km at RPE 2–3 4 km at RPE 3–4 10 km at 95% effort 5 km at RPE 2–3 **Recovery Run** 35:00 at RPE 2–3	**Foundation Run** 5:00 at RPE 2–3 55:00 at RPE 3–4	**Foundation Run** 5:00 at RPE 2–3 1:10:00 at RPE 3–4
14	**Recovery Run** 40:00 at RPE 2–3	**Steady State Run** 5:00 at RPE 2–3 15:00 at RPE 3–4 1:00:00 at RPE 5 20:00 at RPE 2–3 **Recovery Run** 30:00 at RPE 2–3	**Foundation Run** 5:00 at RPE 2–3 55:00 at RPE 3–4	**Foundation Run** 5:00 at RPE 2–3 55:00 at RPE 3–4
15	Rest	**Fartleks** 5:00 at RPE 2–3 15:00 at RPE 3–4 10 × 1:00 at RPE 7–8 / 2:00 at RPE 2–3 20:00 at RPE 3–4	**Foundation Run** 5:00 at RPE 2–3 40:00 at RPE 3–4	**Foundation Run** 5:00 at RPE 2–3 40:00 at RPE 3–4

FRIDAY	SATURDAY	SUNDAY
VO₂max Intervals 5:00 at RPE 2–3 15:00 at RPE 3–4 7 × 2:00 at RPE 7–8* / 2:00 at RPE 2–3 20:00 at RPE 2–3 *Precision Splitting* **Recovery Run** 35:00 at RPE 2–3	**Foundation Run** 5:00 at RPE 2–3 55:00 at RPE 3–4	**Half-Marathon Pace Run** 1 km at RPE 2–3 4 km at RPE 3–4 13 km at HMP 5 km at RPE 2–3
Relaxed 5K Time Trial 1 km at RPE 2–3 4 km at RPE 3–4 5 km at 95% effort 5 km at RPE 2–3 **Recovery Run** 30:00 at RPE 2–3	**Foundation Run** 5:00 at RPE 2–3 55:00 at RPE 3–4	**Endurance Run** 5:00 at RPE 2–3 1:10:00 at RPE 3–4 5:00 at RPE 4–5
Fast Finish Run 5:00 at RPE 2–3 20:00 at RPE 3–4 10:00 at RPE 6	**Foundation Run** 5:00 at RPE 2–3 15:00 at RPE 3–4	**Half-Marathon Race**

12

Marathon Training Plans

The four training plans presented in this chapter are designed to help runners master the art of pacing and find their limit at the marathon distance. The various levels cover the needs of everyone from first-timers to elites. Refer back to Chapter 6 for details on the RPE-based intensity scale used throughout the plans and for full explanations of certain terms and workout types. Online versions of the plans are available for separate purchase on the 80/20 Endurance website. Additionally, device-compatible free versions of the individual workouts can be found at 8020endurance.com/on-pace-workouts.

Marathon

This plan is appropriate for beginning runners preparing for their first marathon event and for more experienced runners who need or prefer a relatively low-volume training program for any reason. Before starting the plan, be sure to build your training to the point where you're comfortably able to run five days a week for up to 10 km.

	MONDAY	TUESDAY	WEDNESDAY	THURSDAY
1	Rest	**Progression Run** 5:00 at RPE 2–3 10:00 at RPE 3–4 8:00 at SSP 4:00 at LTP 2:00 at CV 5:00 at RPE 2–3	**Foundation Run** 5:00 at RPE 2–3 25:00 at RPE 3–4	Rest
2	Rest	**Progression Run** 5:00 at RPE 2–3 20:00 at RPE 3–4 4:00 at LTP 2:00 at CV 1:00 at MAS 5:00 at RPE 2–3	**Foundation Run** 5:00 at RPE 2–3 30:00 at RPE 3–4	Rest
3	Rest	**Progression Run** 5:00 at RPE 2–3 10:00 at RPE 3–4 8:00 at SSP 4:00 at LTP 2:00 at CV 5:00 at RPE 2–3	**Foundation Run** 5:00 at RPE 2–3 25:00 at RPE 3–4	Rest

4	Rest	**Progression Fartleks**
		5:00 at RPE 2–3
		5:00 at RPE 3–4
		2 × (3:00 at RPE 4–5 /
		  1:00 at RPE 2–3)
		2 × (4:00 at RPE 5–6 /
		  1:00 at RPE 2–3)
		10:00 at RPE 2–3
			Foundation Run
			5:00 at RPE 2–3
			30:00 at RPE 3–4
				Rest

5	Rest	**Critical Velocity Intervals** 5:00 at RPE 2–3 5:00 at RPE 3–4 4 × 4:00 at RPE 6–7* / 2:00 at RPE 2–3 10:00 at RPE 2–3 *Precision Splitting*	**Foundation Run** 5:00 at RPE 2–3 35:00 at RPE 3–4	Rest

LEVEL

SSP Steady State Pace
LTP Lactate Threshold Pace
CV Critical Velocity
MAS Maximal Aerobic Speed

5KP 5K Pace

FRIDAY	SATURDAY	SUNDAY
Fartleks 5:00 at RPE 2–3 5:00 at RPE 3–4 4 × 1:00 at RPE 7–8 / 2:00 at RPE 2–3 10:00 at RPE 3–4	**Foundation Run** 5:00 at RPE 2–3 25:00 at RPE 3–4	**Long Run with Fast Finish** 1 km at RPE 2–3 8 km at RPE 3–4 1 km at RPE 4–5
Fartleks 5:00 at RPE 2–3 5:00 at RPE 3–4 6 × 0:20 at RPE 8–9 / 1:40 at RPE 2–3 10:00 at RPE 3–4	**Foundation Run** 5:00 at RPE 2–3 30:00 at RPE 3–4	**Long Run with Fast Finish** 1 km at RPE 2–3 9 km at RPE 3–4 1 km at RPE 4–5
Fartleks 5:00 at RPE 2–3 5:00 at RPE 3–4 6 × 1:00 at RPE 7–8 / 2:00 at RPE 2–3 10:00 at RPE 3–4	**Foundation Run** 5:00 at RPE 2–3 25:00 at RPE 3–4	**Long Run with Fast Finish** 1 km at RPE 2–3 8 km at RPE 3–4 1 km at RPE 4–5
Hill Repetitions 5:00 at RPE 2–3 5:00 at RPE 3–4 8 × 0:30 uphill at RPE 8–9* / 1:30 at RPE 2–3 10:00 at RPE 2–3 *Stretch Intervals*	**Foundation Run** 5:00 at RPE 2–3 30:00 at RPE 3–4	**Long Run with Fast Finish** 1 km at RPE 2–3 11 km at RPE 3–4 1 km at RPE 4–5
Accelerations 5:00 at RPE 2–3 5:00 at RPE 3–4 11:00 acceleration 10:00 at RPE 2–3 3:00 acceleration 10:00 at RPE 2–3	**Foundation Run** 5:00 at RPE 2–3 35:00 at RPE 3–4	**Long Run with Fast Finish** 1 km at RPE 2–3 13 km at RPE 3–4 1 km at RPE 4–5

	MONDAY	**TUESDAY**	**WEDNESDAY**	**THURSDAY**
6	Rest	**Fartleks** 5:00 at RPE 2–3 5:00 at RPE 3–4 1:00 at CV, 1:00 at RPE 2–3 2:00 at LTP, 1:00 at RPE 2–3 3:00 at SSP, 1:00 at RPE 2–3 2:00 at LTP, 1:00 at RPE 2–3 1:00 at CV, 1:00 at RPE 2–3 10:00 at RPE 3–4	**Foundation Run** 5:00 at RPE 2–3 30:00 at RPE 3–4	Rest
7	Rest	**Steady State Run** 5:00 at RPE 2–3 5:00 at RPE 3–4 35:00 at RPE 5 10:00 at RPE 2–3	**Foundation Run** 5:00 at RPE 2–3 35:00 at RPE 3–4	Rest
8	Rest	**Tempo Run** 5:00 at RPE 2–3 5:00 at RPE 3–4 12:00 at RPE 6 5:00 at RPE 2–3 12:00 at RPE 6 10:00 at RPE 2–3	**Foundation Run** 5:00 at RPE 2–3 40:00 at RPE 3–4	Rest
9	Rest	**Fartleks** 5:00 at RPE 2–3 5:00 at RPE 3–4 1:00 at CV, 1:00 at RPE 2–3 2:00 at LTP, 1:00 at RPE 2–3 3:00 at SSP, 1:00 at RPE 2–3 2:00 at LTP, 1:00 at RPE 2–3 1:00 at CV, 1:00 at RPE 2–3 2:00 at LTP, 1:00 at RPE 2–3 1:00 at CV, 1:00 at RPE 2–3 10:00 at RPE 3–4	**Foundation Run** 5:00 at RPE 2–3 35:00 at RPE 3–4	Rest
10	Rest	**Progression Fartleks** 5:00 at RPE 2–3 5:00 at RPE 3–4 2 × (3:00 at RPE 4–5 / 1:00 at RPE 2–3) 2 × (4:00 at RPE 5–6 / 1:00 at RPE 2–3) 2 × (5:00 at RPE 6–7 / 1:00 at RPE 2–3) 10:00 at RPE 2–3	**Foundation Run** 5:00 at RPE 2–3 40:00 at RPE 3–4	Rest
11	Rest	**Critical Velocity Intervals** 5:00 at RPE 2–3 5:00 at RPE 3–4 5 × 4:00 at RPE 6–7* / 2:00 at RPE 2–3 10:00 at RPE 2–3 *Precision Splitting*	**Foundation Run** 5:00 at RPE 2–3 45:00 at RPE 3–4	Rest

FRIDAY	SATURDAY	SUNDAY
Speed Intervals	**Foundation Run**	**Long Run with Fast Finish**
5:00 at RPE 2–3	5:00 at RPE 2–3	1 km at RPE 2–3
5:00 at RPE 3–4	30:00 at RPE 3–4	11 km at RPE 3–4
6 × 0:45 at RPE 8–9* /		1 km at RPE 4–5
1:45 at RPE 2–3		
10:00 at RPE 2–3		
Stretch Intervals		
VO₂max Intervals	**Foundation Run**	**Long Run with Fast Finish**
5:00 at RPE 2–3	5:00 at RPE 2–3	1 km at RPE 2–3
5:00 at RPE 3–4	35:00 at RPE 3–4	15 km at RPE 3–4
4 × 2:00 at RPE 7–8* /		1 km at RPE 4–5
2:00 at RPE 2–3		
10:00 at RPE 2–3		
Precision Splitting		
5K Pace Intervals	**Foundation Run**	**Long Run with Fast Finish**
1 km at RPE 2–3	5:00 at RPE 2–3	1 km at RPE 2–3
1 km at RPE 3–4	40:00 at RPE 3–4	17 km at RPE 3–4
6 × (0.8 km at 5KP* / 1:00 rest)		1 km at RPE 4–5
2 km at RPE 2–3		
Precision Splitting		
Hill Repetitions	**Foundation Run**	**Long Run with Fast Finish**
5:00 at RPE 2–3	5:00 at RPE 2–3	1 km at RPE 2–3
5:00 at RPE 3–4	35:00 at RPE 3–4	13 km at RPE 3–4
6 × 1:00 uphill at RPE 8–9* /		1 km at RPE 4–5
2:00 at RPE 2–3		
10:00 at RPE 2–3		
Stretch Intervals		
5K Pace Intervals	**Foundation Run**	**Long Run with Fast Finish**
1 km at RPE 2–3	5:00 at RPE 2–3	1 km at RPE 2–3
1 km at RPE 3–4	40:00 at RPE 3–4	19 km at RPE 3–4
8 × (0.6 km at 5KP* / 1:00 rest)		1 km at RPE 4–5
2 km at RPE 2–3		
Precision Splitting		
5K Pace Intervals	**Foundation Run**	**Long Run with Fast Finish**
1 km at RPE 2–3	5:00 at RPE 2–3	1 km at RPE 2–3
1 km at RPE 3–4	45:00 at RPE 3–4	21 km at RPE 3–4
8 × (0.6 km at 5KP* / 1:00 rest)		1 km at RPE 4–5
2 km at RPE 2–3		
Precision Splitting		

Marathon

	MONDAY	TUESDAY	WEDNESDAY	THURSDAY
12	Rest	**Fartleks** 5:00 at RPE 2–3 5:00 at RPE 3–4 1:00 at CV, 1:00 at RPE 2–3 2:00 at LTP, 1:00 at RPE 2–3 3:00 at SSP, 1:00 at RPE 2–3 2:00 at LTP, 1:00 at RPE 2–3 1:00 at CV, 1:00 at RPE 2–3 2:00 at LTP, 1:00 at RPE 2–3 1:00 at CV, 1:00 at RPE 2–3 2:00 at LTP, 1:00 at RPE 2–3 3:00 at SSP, 1:00 at RPE 2–3 10:00 at RPE 3–4	**Foundation Run** 5:00 at RPE 2–3 40:00 at RPE 3–4	Rest
13	Rest	**Steady State Run** 5:00 at RPE 2–3 5:00 at RPE 3–4 40:00 at RPE 5 10:00 at RPE 2–3	**Foundation Run** 5:00 at RPE 2–3 45:00 at RPE 3–4	Rest
14	Rest	**Tempo Run** 5:00 at RPE 2–3 5:00 at RPE 3–4 14:00 at RPE 6 5:00 at RPE 2–3 14:00 at RPE 6 10:00 at RPE 2–3	**Foundation Run** 5:00 at RPE 2–3 50:00 at RPE 3–4	Rest
15	Rest	**Progression Run** 5:00 at RPE 2–3 15:00 at RPE 3–4 12:00 at SSP 6:00 at LTP 3:00 at CV 5:00 at RPE 2–3	**Foundation Run** 5:00 at RPE 2–3 40:00 at RPE 3–4	Rest
16	Rest	**Steady State Run** 5:00 at RPE 2–3 5:00 at RPE 3–4 50:00 at RPE 5 10:00 at RPE 2–3	**Foundation Run** 5:00 at RPE 2–3 50:00 at RPE 3–4	Rest
17	Rest	**Relaxed 10K Time Trial** 1 km at RPE 2–3 1 km at RPE 3–4 10 km at 95% effort 2 km at RPE 2–3	**Foundation Run** 5:00 at RPE 2–3 40:00 at RPE 3–4	Rest
18	Rest	**Fartleks** 5:00 at RPE 2–3 5:00 at RPE 3–4 6 × 1:00 at RPE 7–8 / 2:00 at RPE 2–3 10:00 at RPE 3–4	**Foundation Run** 5:00 at RPE 2–3 40:00 at RPE 3–4	Rest

FRIDAY	SATURDAY	SUNDAY
Speed Intervals 5:00 at RPE 2–3 5:00 at RPE 3–4 8 × 0:45 at RPE 8–9* / 1:45 at RPE 2–3 10:00 at RPE 2–3 *Stretch Intervals*	**Foundation Run** 5:00 at RPE 2–3 40:00 at RPE 3–4	**Long Run with Fast Finish** 1 km at RPE 2–3 15 km at RPE 3–4 1 km at RPE 4–5
Accelerations 5:00 at RPE 2–3 5:00 at RPE 3–4 11:00 acceleration 10:00 at RPE 2–3 6:00 acceleration 10:00 at RPE 2–3	**Foundation Run** 5:00 at RPE 2–3 45:00 at RPE 3–4	**Long Run with Fast Finish** 1 km at RPE 2–3 23 km at RPE 3–4 1 km at RPE 4–5
Hill Repetitions 5:00 at RPE 2–3 5:00 at RPE 3–4 5 × 2:00 uphill at RPE 7–8* / 1:00 at RPE 2–3 10:00 at RPE 2–3 *Precision Splitting*	**Foundation Run** 5:00 at RPE 2–3 50:00 at RPE 3–4	**Long Run with Fast Finish** 1 km at RPE 2–3 25 km at RPE 3–4 1 km at RPE 4–5
Speed Intervals 5:00 at RPE 2–3 5:00 at RPE 3–4 10 × 0:45 at RPE 8–9* / 1:45 at RPE 2–3 10:00 at RPE 2–3 *Stretch Intervals*	**Foundation Run** 5:00 at RPE 2–3 40:00 at RPE 3–4	**Long Run with Fast Finish** 1 km at RPE 2–3 17 km at RPE 3–4 1 km at RPE 4–5
Relaxed 5K Time Trial 1 km at RPE 2–3 1 km at RPE 3–4 5 km at 95% effort 2 km at RPE 2–3	**Foundation Run** 5:00 at RPE 2–3 50:00 at RPE 3–4	**Long Run with Fast Finish** 1 km at RPE 2–3 27 km at RPE 3–4 1 km at RPE 4–5
VO₂max Intervals 5:00 at RPE 2–3 5:00 at RPE 3–4 4 × 2:00 at RPE 7–8* / 2:00 at RPE 2–3 10:00 at RPE 2–3 *Precision Splitting*	**Foundation Run** 5:00 at RPE 2–3 40:00 at RPE 3–4	**Long Run with Fast Finish** 1 km at RPE 2–3 15 km at RPE 3–4 1 km at RPE 4–5
Fast Finish Run 5:00 at RPE 2–3 15:00 at RPE 3–4 10:00 at RPE 6	**Foundation Run** 5:00 at RPE 2–3 15:00 at RPE 3–4	**Marathon Race**

Marathon

Marathon

This plan is designed for runners who are ready to take their training load up a notch in order to improve their marathon time. Before starting the plan, be sure to build your training to the point where you're comfortably able to run six days a week for up to 12 km.

	MONDAY	TUESDAY	WEDNESDAY	THURSDAY
1	Rest	**Progression Run** 5:00 at RPE 2–3 15:00 at RPE 3–4 8:00 at SSP 4:00 at LTP 2:00 at CV 5:00 at RPE 2–3	**Foundation Run** 5:00 at RPE 2–3 25:00 at RPE 3–4	**Foundation Run** 5:00 at RPE 2–3 25:00 at RPE 3–4
2	Rest	**Progression Run** 5:00 at RPE 2–3 25:00 at RPE 3–4 4:00 at LTP 2:00 at CV 1:00 at MAS 5:00 at RPE 2–3	**Foundation Run** 5:00 at RPE 2–3 30:00 at RPE 3–4	**Foundation Run** 5:00 at RPE 2–3 30:00 at RPE 3–4
3	Rest	**Progression Run** 5:00 at RPE 2–3 10:00 at RPE 3–4 8:00 at SSP 4:00 at LTP 2:00 at CV 5:00 at RPE 2–3	**Foundation Run** 5:00 at RPE 2–3 25:00 at RPE 3–4	**Foundation Run** 5:00 at RPE 2–3 25:00 at RPE 3–4

4	Rest	**Progression Fartleks**
		5:00 at RPE 2–3
		5:00 at RPE 3–4
		2 × (3:00 at RPE 4–5 /
		  1:00 at RPE 2–3)
		2 × (4:00 at RPE 5–6 /
		  1:00 at RPE 2–3)
		10:00 at RPE 2–3
			Foundation Run
			5:00 at RPE 2–3
			30:00 at RPE 3–4
				Foundation Run
				5:00 at RPE 2–3
				30:00 at RPE 3–4

5	Rest	**Critical Velocity Intervals** 5:00 at RPE 2–3 5:00 at RPE 3–4 5 × 4:00 at RPE 6–7* / 2:00 at RPE 2–3 10:00 at RPE 2–3 *Precision Splitting*	**Foundation Run** 5:00 at RPE 2–3 35:00 at RPE 3–4	**Foundation Run** 5:00 at RPE 2–3 35:00 at RPE 3–4

LEVEL

SSP Steady State Pace
LTP Lactate Threshold Pace
CV Critical Velocity
MAS Maximal Aerobic Speed

5KP 5K Pace
MP Marathon Pace

FRIDAY	SATURDAY	SUNDAY
Fartleks 5:00 at RPE 2–3 5:00 at RPE 3–4 6 × 1:00 at RPE 7–8 / 2:00 at RPE 2–3 10:00 at RPE 3–4	**Foundation Run** 5:00 at RPE 2–3 25:00 at RPE 3–4	**Long Run with Fast Finish** 1 km at RPE 2–3 11 km at RPE 3–4 1 km at RPE 4–5
Fartleks 5:00 at RPE 2–3 5:00 at RPE 3–4 6 × 0:20 at RPE 8–9 / 1:40 at RPE 2–3 10:00 at RPE 3–4	**Foundation Run** 5:00 at RPE 2–3 30:00 at RPE 3–4	**Long Run with Fast Finish** 1 km at RPE 2–3 13 km at RPE 3–4 1 km at RPE 4–5
Fartleks 5:00 at RPE 2–3 5:00 at RPE 3–4 6 × 1:00 at RPE 7–8 / 2:00 at RPE 2–3 10:00 at RPE 3–4	**Foundation Run** 5:00 at RPE 2–3 25:00 at RPE 3–4	**Long Run with Fast Finish** 1 km at RPE 2–3 11 km at RPE 3–4 1 km at RPE 4–5
Hill Repetitions 5:00 at RPE 2–3 5:00 at RPE 3–4 8 × 0:30 uphill at RPE 8–9* / 1:30 at RPE 2–3 10:00 at RPE 2–3 *Stretch Intervals	**Foundation Run** 5:00 at RPE 2–3 30:00 at RPE 3–4	**Long Run with Fast Finish** 1 km at RPE 2–3 15 km at RPE 3–4 1 km at RPE 4–5
Accelerations 5:00 at RPE 2–3 5:00 at RPE 3–4 11:00 acceleration 10:00 at RPE 2–3 6:00 acceleration 10:00 at RPE 2–3	**Foundation Run** 5:00 at RPE 2–3 35:00 at RPE 3–4	**Long Run with Fast Finish** 1 km at RPE 2–3 17 km at RPE 3–4 1 km at RPE 4–5

	MONDAY	TUESDAY	WEDNESDAY	THURSDAY
6	Rest	**Fartleks** 5:00 at RPE 2–3 5:00 at RPE 3–4 1:00 at CV, 1:00 at RPE 2–3 2:00 at LTP, 1:00 at RPE 2–3 3:00 at SSP, 1:00 at RPE 2–3 2:00 at LTP, 1:00 at RPE 2–3 1:00 at CV, 1:00 at RPE 2–3 2:00 at LTP, 1:00 at RPE 2–3 3:00 at SSP, 1:00 at RPE 2–3 10:00 at RPE 3–4	**Foundation Run** 5:00 at RPE 2–3 30:00 at RPE 3–4	**Foundation Run** 5:00 at RPE 2–3 30:00 at RPE 3–4
7	Rest	**Steady State Run** 5:00 at RPE 2–3 5:00 at RPE 3–4 40:00 at RPE 5 10:00 at RPE 2–3	**Foundation Run** 5:00 at RPE 2–3 35:00 at RPE 3–4	**Foundation Run** 5:00 at RPE 2–3 35:00 at RPE 3–4
8	Rest	**Tempo Run** 5:00 at RPE 2–3 5:00 at RPE 3–4 14:00 at RPE 6 5:00 at RPE 2–3 14:00 at RPE 6 10:00 at RPE 2–3	**Foundation Run** 5:00 at RPE 2–3 40:00 at RPE 3–4	**Foundation Run** 5:00 at RPE 2–3 40:00 at RPE 3–4
9	Rest	**Progression Run** 5:00 at RPE 2–3 20:00 at RPE 3–4 8:00 at LTP 4:00 at CV 2:00 at MAS 5:00 at RPE 2–3	**Foundation Run** 5:00 at RPE 2–3 35:00 at RPE 3–4	**Foundation Run** 5:00 at RPE 2–3 35:00 at RPE 3–4

10	Rest	**Progression Fartleks**
		5:00 at RPE 2–3
		5:00 at RPE 3–4
		2 × (3:00 at RPE 4–5 /
		  1:00 at RPE 2–3)
		2 × (4:00 at RPE 5–6 /
		  1:00 at RPE 2–3)
		2 × (5:00 at RPE 6–7 /
		  1:00 at RPE 2–3)
		10:00 at RPE 2–3
			Foundation Run
			5:00 at RPE 2–3
			40:00 at RPE 3–4
				Foundation Run
				5:00 at RPE 2–3
				40:00 at RPE 3–4

11	Rest	**Critical Velocity Intervals** 5:00 at RPE 2–3 5:00 at RPE 3–4 6 × 4:00 at RPE 6–7* / 2:00 at RPE 2–3 10:00 at RPE 2–3 *Precision Splitting*	**Foundation Run** 5:00 at RPE 2–3 45:00 at RPE 3–4	**Foundation Run** 5:00 at RPE 2–3 45:00 at RPE 3–4

ON PACE

FRIDAY	SATURDAY	SUNDAY
Speed Intervals 5:00 at RPE 2–3 5:00 at RPE 3–4 8 × 0:45 at RPE 8–9* / 1:45 at RPE 2–3 10:00 at RPE 2–3 *Stretch Intervals*	**Foundation Run** 5:00 at RPE 2–3 30:00 at RPE 3–4	**Long Run with Fast Finish** 1 km at RPE 2–3 11 km at RPE 3–4 1 km at RPE 4–5
VO₂max Intervals 5:00 at RPE 2–3 5:00 at RPE 3–4 5 × 2:00 at RPE 7–8* / 2:00 at RPE 2–3 10:00 at RPE 2–3 *Precision Splitting*	**Foundation Run** 5:00 at RPE 2–3 35:00 at RPE 3–4	**Long Run with Fast Finish** 1 km at RPE 2–3 19 km at RPE 3–4 1 km at RPE 4–5
5K Pace Intervals 1 km at RPE 2–3 1 km at RPE 3–4 6 × (0.8 km at 5KP* / 1:00 rest) 2 km at RPE 2–3 *Precision Splitting*	**Foundation Run** 5:00 at RPE 2–3 40:00 at RPE 3–4	**Long Run with Fast Finish** 1 km at RPE 2–3 21 km at RPE 3–4 1 km at RPE 4–5
Hill Repetitions 5:00 at RPE 2–3 5:00 at RPE 3–4 8 × 1:00 uphill at RPE 8–9* / 2:00 at RPE 2–3 10:00 at RPE 2–3 *Stretch Intervals*	**Foundation Run** 5:00 at RPE 2–3 35:00 at RPE 3–4	**Long Run with Fast Finish** 1 km at RPE 2–3 13 km at RPE 3–4 1 km at RPE 4–5
The Prefontaine 1 km at RPE 2–3 1 km at RPE 3–4 ? × 200m at RPE 9 / 200m at RPE 6 1 km at RPE 2–3 1 km at RPE 3–4 *(? = Go to failure)*	**Foundation Run** 5:00 at RPE 2–3 40:00 at RPE 3–4	**Long Run with Fast Finish** 1 km at RPE 2–3 23 km at RPE 3–4 1 km at RPE 4–5
VO₂max Intervals 5:00 at RPE 2–3 5:00 at RPE 3–4 6 × 2:00 at RPE 7–8* / 2:00 at RPE 2–3 10:00 at RPE 2–3 *Precision Splitting*	**Foundation Run** 5:00 at RPE 2–3 45:00 at RPE 3–4	**Long Run with Fast Finish** 1 km at RPE 2–3 25 km at RPE 3–4 1 km at RPE 4–5

Marathon

1

	MONDAY	TUESDAY	WEDNESDAY	THURSDAY
12	Rest	**Fartleks** 5:00 at RPE 2–3 5:00 at RPE 3–4 1:00 at CV, 1:00 at RPE 2–3 2:00 at LTP, 1:00 at RPE 2–3 3:00 at SSP, 1:00 at RPE 2–3 2:00 at LTP, 1:00 at RPE 2–3 1:00 at CV, 1:00 at RPE 2–3 2:00 at LTP, 1:00 at RPE 2–3 1:00 at CV, 1:00 at RPE 2–3 2:00 at LTP, 1:00 at RPE 2–3 3:00 at SSP, 1:00 at RPE 2–3 10:00 at RPE 3–4	**Foundation Run** 5:00 at RPE 2–3 40:00 at RPE 3–4	**Foundation Run** 5:00 at RPE 2–3 40:00 at RPE 3–4
13	Rest	**Steady State Run** 5:00 at RPE 2–3 5:00 at RPE 3–4 45:00 at RPE 5 10:00 at RPE 2–3	**Foundation Run** 5:00 at RPE 2–3 45:00 at RPE 3–4	**Foundation Run** 5:00 at RPE 2–3 45:00 at RPE 3–4
14	Rest	**Tempo Run** 5:00 at RPE 2–3 5:00 at RPE 3–4 14:00 at RPE 6 5:00 at RPE 2–3 14:00 at RPE 6 10:00 at RPE 2–3	**Foundation Run** 5:00 at RPE 2–3 50:00 at RPE 3–4	**Foundation Run** 5:00 at RPE 2–3 50:00 at RPE 3–4
15	Rest	**Progression Run** 5:00 at RPE 2–3 15:00 at RPE 3–4 12:00 at SSP 6:00 at LTP 3:00 at CV 5:00 at RPE 2–3	**Foundation Run** 5:00 at RPE 2–3 40:00 at RPE 3–4	**Foundation Run** 5:00 at RPE 2–3 40:00 at RPE 3–4
16	Rest	**Steady State Run** 5:00 at RPE 2–3 5:00 at RPE 3–4 50:00 at RPE 5 10:00 at RPE 2–3	**Foundation Run** 5:00 at RPE 2–3 50:00 at RPE 3–4	**Foundation Run** 5:00 at RPE 2–3 50:00 at RPE 3–4
17	Rest	**Relaxed 10K Time Trial** 1 km at RPE 2–3 1 km at RPE 3–4 10 km at 95% effort 2 km at RPE 2–3	**Foundation Run** 5:00 at RPE 2–3 40:00 at RPE 3–4	**Foundation Run** 5:00 at RPE 2–3 40:00 at RPE 3–4
18	Rest	**Fartleks** 5:00 at RPE 2–3 5:00 at RPE 3–4 6 × 1:00 at RPE 7–8 / 2:00 at RPE 2–3 10:00 at RPE 3–4	**Foundation Run** 5:00 at RPE 2–3 40:00 at RPE 3–4	**Foundation Run** 5:00 at RPE 2–3 35:00 at RPE 3–4

FRIDAY	SATURDAY	SUNDAY
Speed Intervals 5:00 at RPE 2–3 5:00 at RPE 3–4 10 × 0:45 at RPE 8–9* / 1:45 at RPE 2–3 10:00 at RPE 2–3 *Stretch Intervals*	**Foundation Run** 5:00 at RPE 2–3 40:00 at RPE 3–4	**Long Run with Fast Finish** 1 km at RPE 2–3 15 km at RPE 3–4 1 km at RPE 4–5
5K Pace Intervals 1 km at RPE 2–3 1 km at RPE 3–4 8 × (0.6 km at 5KP* / 1:00 rest) 2 km at RPE 2–3 *Precision Splitting*	**Foundation Run** 5:00 at RPE 2–3 45:00 at RPE 3–4	**Long Run with Fast Finish** 1 km at RPE 2–3 27 km at RPE 3–4 1 km at RPE 4–5
Relaxed 5K Time Trial 1 km at RPE 2–3 1 km at RPE 3–4 5 km at 95% effort 2 km at RPE 2–3	**Foundation Run** 5:00 at RPE 2–3 50:00 at RPE 3–4	**Long Run with Fast Finish** 1 km at RPE 2–3 29 km at RPE 3–4 1 km at RPE 4–5
Hill Repetitions 5:00 at RPE 2–3 5:00 at RPE 3–4 4 × 2:00 uphill at RPE 7–8* / 2:00 at RPE 2–3 10:00 at RPE 2–3 *Stretch Intervals*	**Foundation Run** 5:00 at RPE 2–3 40:00 at RPE 3–4	**Long Run with Fast Finish** 1 km at RPE 2–3 17 km at RPE 3–4 1 km at RPE 4–5
Speed Intervals 5:00 at RPE 2–3 5:00 at RPE 3–4 8 × 1:00 at RPE 8–9* / 2:00 at RPE 2–3 10:00 at RPE 2–3 *Stretch Intervals*	**Foundation Run** 5:00 at RPE 2–3 50:00 at RPE 3–4	**Marathon Pace Run** 1 km (0.6 mile) at RPE 2–3 2 km (1.2 miles) at RPE 3–4 20 km (12.4 miles) at MP 2 km (1.2 miles) at RPE 2–3
VO$_2$max Intervals 5:00 at RPE 2–3 5:00 at RPE 3–4 5 × 2:00 at RPE 7–8* / 2:00 at RPE 2–3 10:00 at RPE 2–3 *Precision Splitting*	**Foundation Run** 5:00 at RPE 2–3 40:00 at RPE 3–4	**Long Run with Fast Finish** 1 km at RPE 2–3 15 km at RPE 3–4 1 km at RPE 4–5
Fast Finish Run 5:00 at RPE 2–3 15:00 at RPE 3–4 10:00 at RPE 6	**Foundation Run** 5:00 at RPE 2–3 15:00 at RPE 3–4	**Marathon Race**

Marathon

This plan is a good fit for experienced competitive runners who are prepared to train hard in pursuit of improved marathon performance. Before starting the plan, be sure to build your training to the point where you're comfortably able to run seven days a week for up to 17 km.

	MONDAY	TUESDAY	WEDNESDAY	THURSDAY
1	**Recovery Run** 30:00 at RPE 2–3	**Progression Run** 5:00 at RPE 2–3 25:00 at RPE 3–4 8:00 at SSP 4:00 at LTP 2:00 at CV 5:00 at RPE 2–3	**Foundation Run** 5:00 at RPE 2–3 40:00 at RPE 3–4	**Foundation Run** 5:00 at RPE 2–3 40:00 at RPE 3–4
2	**Recovery Run** 30:00 at RPE 2–3	**Progression Run** 5:00 at RPE 2–3 35:00 at RPE 3–4 4:00 at LTP 2:00 at CV 1:00 at MAS 5:00 at RPE 2–3	**Foundation Run** 5:00 at RPE 2–3 45:00 at RPE 3–4	**Foundation Run** 5:00 at RPE 2–3 45:00 at RPE 3–4
3	Rest	**Progression Run** 5:00 at RPE 2–3 25:00 at RPE 3–4 8:00 at SSP 4:00 at LTP 2:00 at CV 5:00 at RPE 2–3	**Foundation Run** 5:00 at RPE 2–3 40:00 at RPE 3–4	**Foundation Run** 5:00 at RPE 2–3 40:00 at RPE 3–4
4	**Recovery Run** 30:00 at RPE 2–3	**Progression Fartleks** 5:00 at RPE 2–3 5:00 at RPE 3–4 2 × (3:00 at RPE 4–5 / 1:00 at RPE 2–3) 2 × (4:00 at RPE 5–6 / 1:00 at RPE 2–3) 2 × (5:00 at RPE 6–7 / 1:00 at RPE 2–3) 15:00 at RPE 2–3	**Foundation Run** 5:00 at RPE 2–3 45:00 at RPE 3–4	**Foundation Run** 5:00 at RPE 2–3 45:00 at RPE 3–4
5	**Recovery Run** 30:00 at RPE 2–3	**Critical Velocity Intervals** 5:00 at RPE 2–3 10:00 at RPE 3–4 6 × 4:00 at RPE 6–7* / 2:00 at RPE 2–3 15:00 at RPE 2–3 *Precision Splitting*	**Foundation Run** 5:00 at RPE 2–3 50:00 at RPE 3–4	**Foundation Run** 5:00 at RPE 2–3 50:00 at RPE 3–4

LEVEL

SSP Steady State Pace
LTP Lactate Threshold Pace
CV Critical Velocity
MAS Maximal Aerobic Speed

5KP 5K Pace
MP Marathon Pace

FRIDAY	SATURDAY	SUNDAY
Fartleks 5:00 at RPE 2–3 10:00 at RPE 3–4 8 × 1:00 at RPE 7–8 / 2:00 at RPE 2–3 15:00 at RPE 3–4	**Foundation Run** 5:00 at RPE 2–3 40:00 at RPE 3–4	**Long Run with Fast Finish** 1 km at RPE 2–3 15 km at RPE 3–4 1 km at RPE 4–5
Fartleks 5:00 at RPE 2–3 10:00 at RPE 3–4 8 × 0:20 at RPE 8–9 / 1:40 at RPE 2–3 15:00 at RPE 3–4	**Foundation Run** 5:00 at RPE 2–3 45:00 at RPE 3–4	**Long Run with Fast Finish** 1 km at RPE 2–3 17 km at RPE 3–4 1 km at RPE 4–5
Fartleks 5:00 at RPE 2–3 10:00 at RPE 3–4 8 × 1:00 at RPE 7–8 / 2:00 at RPE 2–3 15:00 at RPE 3–4	**Foundation Run** 5:00 at RPE 2–3 40:00 at RPE 3–4	**Long Run with Fast Finish** 1 km at RPE 2–3 15 km at RPE 3–4 1 km at RPE 4–5
Hill Repetitions 5:00 at RPE 2–3 10:00 at RPE 3–4 10 × 0:30 uphill at RPE 8–9* / 1:30 at RPE 2–3 15:00 at RPE 2–3 *Stretch Intervals	**Foundation Run** 5:00 at RPE 2–3 45:00 at RPE 3–4	**Long Run with Fast Finish** 1 km at RPE 2–3 21 km at RPE 3–4 1 km at RPE 4–5
Accelerations 5:00 at RPE 2–3 10:00 at RPE 3–4 11:00 acceleration 10:00 at RPE 2–3 6:00 acceleration 10:00 at RPE 2–3	**Foundation Run** 5:00 at RPE 2–3 50:00 at RPE 3–4	**Long Run with Fast Finish** 1 km at RPE 2–3 25 km at RPE 3–4 1 km at RPE 4–5

	MONDAY	TUESDAY	WEDNESDAY	THURSDAY
6	Rest	**Fartleks** 5:00 at RPE 2–3 10:00 at RPE 3–4 1:00 at CV, 1:00 at RPE 2–3 2:00 at LTP, 1:00 at RPE 2–3 3:00 at SSP, 1:00 at RPE 2–3 2:00 at LTP, 1:00 at RPE 2–3 1:00 at CV, 1:00 at RPE 2–3 2:00 at LTP, 1:00 at RPE 2–3 3:00 at SSP, 1:00 at RPE 2–3 15:00 at RPE 3–4	**Foundation Run** 5:00 at RPE 2–3 45:00 at RPE 3–4	**Foundation Run** 5:00 at RPE 2–3 45:00 at RPE 3–4
7	**Recovery Run** 30:00 at RPE 2–3	**Steady State Run** 5:00 at RPE 2–3 10:00 at RPE 3–4 45:00 at RPE 5 15:00 at RPE 2–3	**Foundation Run** 5:00 at RPE 2–3 50:00 at RPE 3–4	**Foundation Run** 5:00 at RPE 2–3 50:00 at RPE 3–4
8	**Recovery Run** 30:00 at RPE 2–3	**Tempo Run** 5:00 at RPE 2–3 10:00 at RPE 3–4 16:00 at RPE 6 5:00 at RPE 2–3 16:00 at RPE 6 15:00 at RPE 2–3	**Foundation Run** 5:00 at RPE 2–3 55:00 at RPE 3–4	**Foundation Run** 5:00 at RPE 2–3 55:00 at RPE 3–4
9	Rest	**Progression Run** 5:00 at RPE 2–3 35:00 at RPE 3–4 8:00 at LTP 4:00 at CV 2:00 at MAS 5:00 at RPE 2–3	**Foundation Run** 5:00 at RPE 2–3 45:00 at RPE 3–4	**Foundation Run** 5:00 at RPE 2–3 45:00 at RPE 3–4

10	**Recovery Run**
	30:00 at RPE 2–3
		Progression Fartleks
		5:00 at RPE 2–3
		10:00 at RPE 3–4
		2 × (3:00 at RPE 4–5 /
		  1:00 at RPE 2–3)
		2 × (4:00 at RPE 5–6 /
		  1:00 at RPE 2–3)
		2 × (5:00 at RPE 6–7 /
		  1:00 at RPE 2–3)
		2 × (6:00 at RPE 7–8 /
		  1:00 at RPE 2–3)
		15:00 at RPE 2–3
			Foundation Run
			5:00 at RPE 2–3
			55:00 at RPE 3–4
				Foundation Run
				5:00 at RPE 2–3
				55:00 at RPE 3–4

11	**Recovery Run** 30:00 at RPE 2–3	**Critical Velocity Intervals** 5:00 at RPE 2–3 10:00 at RPE 3–4 7 × 4:00 at RPE 6–7* / 2:00 at RPE 2–3 15:00 at RPE 2–3 *Precision Splitting*	**Foundation Run** 5:00 at RPE 2–3 55:00 at RPE 3–4	**Foundation Run** 5:00 at RPE 2–3 55:00 at RPE 3–4

FRIDAY	SATURDAY	SUNDAY
Speed Intervals 5:00 at RPE 2–3 10:00 at RPE 3–4 10 × 0:45 at RPE 8–9* / 1:45 at RPE 2–3 15:00 at RPE 2–3 *Stretch Intervals*	**Foundation Run** 5:00 at RPE 2–3 45:00 at RPE 3–4	**Long Run with Fast Finish** 1 km at RPE 2–3 17 km at RPE 3–4 1 km at RPE 4–5
VO₂max Intervals 5:00 at RPE 2–3 10:00 at RPE 3–4 6 × 2:00 at RPE 7–8* / 2:00 at RPE 2–3 15:00 at RPE 2–3 *Precision Splitting*	**Foundation Run** 5:00 at RPE 2–3 50:00 at RPE 3–4	**Depletion Run** 5:00 at RPE 2–3 1:55:00 at RPE 3–4 *No calories before or during*
5K Pace Intervals 1 km at RPE 2–3 2.5 km at RPE 3–4 6 × (0.8 km at 5KP* / 1:00 rest) 3.5 km at RPE 2–3 *Precision Splitting*	**Foundation Run** 5:00 at RPE 2–3 55:00 at RPE 3–4	**Marathon Pace Run** 1 km (0.6 mile) at RPE 2–3 2 km (1.2 miles) at RPE 3–4 6 × 1.5 km (0.9 mile) at MP / 1.5 km (0.9 mile) at RPE 3–4 2 km (1.2 miles) at RPE 2–3
Hill Repetitions 5:00 at RPE 2–3 10:00 at RPE 3–4 8 × 1:00 uphill at RPE 8–9* / 2:00 at RPE 2–3 15:00 at RPE 2–3 *Stretch Intervals*	**Foundation Run** 5:00 at RPE 2–3 45:00 at RPE 3–4	**Long Run with Fast Finish** 1 km at RPE 2–3 19 km at RPE 3–4 1 km at RPE 4–5
The Prefontaine 1 km at RPE 2–3 2.5 km at RPE 3–4 ? × 200m at RPE 9 / 200m at RPE 6 1 km at RPE 2–3 2.5 km at RPE 3–4 *(? = Go to failure)*	**Foundation Run** 5:00 at RPE 2–3 55:00 at RPE 3–4	**Long Run with Fast Finish** 1 km at RPE 2–3 29 km at RPE 3–4 1 km at RPE 4–5
VO₂max Intervals 5:00 at RPE 2–3 10:00 at RPE 3–4 7 × 2:00 at RPE 7–8* / 2:00 at RPE 2–3 15:00 at RPE 2–3 *Precision Splitting*	**Foundation Run** 5:00 at RPE 2–3 55:00 at RPE 3–4	**Marathon Pace Run** 1 km (0.6 mile) at RPE 2–3 2 km (1.2 miles) at RPE 3–4 20 km (12.4 miles) at MP 2 km (1.2 miles) at RPE 2–3

Marathon

2

	MONDAY	TUESDAY	WEDNESDAY	THURSDAY
12	Rest	**Fartleks** 5:00 at RPE 2–3 10:00 at RPE 3–4 1:00 at CV, 1:00 at RPE 2–3 2:00 at LTP, 1:00 at RPE 2–3 3:00 at SSP, 1:00 at RPE 2–3 2:00 at LTP, 1:00 at RPE 2–3 1:00 at CV, 1:00 at RPE 2–3 2:00 at LTP, 1:00 at RPE 2–3 3:00 at SSP, 1:00 at RPE 2–3 2:00 at LTP, 1:00 at RPE 2–3 1:00 at CV, 1:00 at RPE 2–3 15:00 at RPE 3–4	**Foundation Run** 5:00 at RPE 2–3 50:00 at RPE 3–4	**Foundation Run** 5:00 at RPE 2–3 50:00 at RPE 3–4
13	**Recovery Run** 30:00 at RPE 2–3	**Steady State Run** 5:00 at RPE 2–3 10:00 at RPE 3–4 50:00 at RPE 5 15:00 at RPE 2–3	**Foundation Run** 5:00 at RPE 2–3 55:00 at RPE 3–4	**Foundation Run** 5:00 at RPE 2–3 55:00 at RPE 3–4
14	**Recovery Run** 30:00 at RPE 2–3	**Tempo Run** 5:00 at RPE 2–3 10:00 at RPE 3–4 20:00 at RPE 6 5:00 at RPE 2–3 20:00 at RPE 6 15:00 at RPE 2–3	**Foundation Run** 5:00 at RPE 2–3 55:00 at RPE 3–4	**Foundation Run** 5:00 at RPE 2–3 55:00 at RPE 3–4
15	Rest	**Progression Run** 5:00 at RPE 2–3 25:00 at RPE 3–4 12:00 at SSP 6:00 at LTP 3:00 at CV 5:00 at RPE 2–3	**Foundation Run** 5:00 at RPE 2–3 50:00 at RPE 3–4	**Foundation Run** 5:00 at RPE 2–3 50:00 at RPE 3–4
16	**Recovery Run** 30:00 at RPE 2–3	**Steady State Run** 5:00 at RPE 2–3 10:00 at RPE 3–4 55:00 at RPE 5 15:00 at RPE 2–3	**Foundation Run** 5:00 at RPE 2–3 55:00 at RPE 3–4	**Foundation Run** 5:00 at RPE 2–3 55:00 at RPE 3–4
17	**Recovery Run** 30:00 at RPE 2–3	**Relaxed 10K Time Trial** 1 km at RPE 2–3 2.5 km at RPE 3–4 10 km at 95% effort 3.5 km at RPE 2–3	**Foundation Run** 5:00 at RPE 2–3 55:00 at RPE 3–4	**Foundation Run** 5:00 at RPE 2–3 50:00 at RPE 3–4
18	Rest	**Fartleks** 5:00 at RPE 2–3 10:00 at RPE 3–4 8 × 1:00 at RPE 7–8 / 2:00 at RPE 2–3 15:00 at RPE 3–4	**Foundation Run** 5:00 at RPE 2–3 40:00 at RPE 3–4	**Foundation Run** 5:00 at RPE 2–3 35:00 at RPE 3–4

FRIDAY	SATURDAY	SUNDAY
Speed Intervals 5:00 at RPE 2–3 10:00 at RPE 3–4 10 × 0:45 at RPE 8–9* / 1:45 at RPE 2–3 15:00 at RPE 2–3 *Stretch Intervals*	**Foundation Run** 5:00 at RPE 2–3 50:00 at RPE 3–4	**Depletion Run** 5:00 at RPE 2–3 2:15:00 at RPE 3–4 *No calories before or during*
5K Pace Intervals 1 km at RPE 2–3 2.5 km at RPE 3–4 8 × (0.6 km at 5KP* / 1:00 rest) 3.5 km at RPE 2–3 *Precision Splitting*	**Foundation Run** 5:00 at RPE 2–3 55:00 at RPE 3–4	**Long Run with Fast Finish** 1 km at RPE 2–3 30 km at RPE 3–4 2 km at RPE 5–6* *Note the slightly more aggressive fast finish.*
Relaxed 5K Time Trial 1 km at RPE 2–3 2.5 km at RPE 3–4 5 km at 95% effort 3.5 km at RPE 2–3	**Foundation Run** 5:00 at RPE 2–3 55:00 at RPE 3–4	**Long Run with Fast Finish** 1 km at RPE 2–3 32 km at RPE 3–4 2 km at RPE 5–6* *Note the slightly more aggressive fast finish.*
Hill Repetitions 5:00 at RPE 2–3 10:00 at RPE 3–4 5 × 2:00 uphill at RPE 7–8* / 2:00 at RPE 2–3 15:00 at RPE 2–3 *Stretch Intervals*	**Foundation Run** 5:00 at RPE 2–3 50:00 at RPE 3–4	**Depletion Run** 5:00 at RPE 2–3 2:35:00 at RPE 3–4 *No calories before or during*
Speed Intervals 5:00 at RPE 2–3 10:00 at RPE 3–4 8 × 1:00 at RPE 8–9* / 2:00 at RPE 2–3 15:00 at RPE 2–3 *Stretch Intervals*	**Foundation Run** 5:00 at RPE 2–3 55:00 at RPE 3–4	**Marathon Pace Run** 1 km (0.6 mile) at RPE 2–3 2 km (1.2 miles) at RPE 3–4 26 km (16.1 miles) at MP 2 km (1.2 miles) at RPE 2–3
VO$_2$max Intervals 5:00 at RPE 2–3 10:00 at RPE 3–4 6 × 2:00 at RPE 7–8* / 2:00 at RPE 2–3 15:00 at RPE 2–3 *Precision Splitting*	**Foundation Run** 5:00 at RPE 2–3 45:00 at RPE 3–4	**Long Run with Fast Finish** 1 km at RPE 2–3 16 km at RPE 3–4 2 km at RPE 5–6* *Note the slightly more aggressive fast finish.*
Fast Finish Run 5:00 at RPE 2–3 20:00 at RPE 3–4 10:00 at RPE 6	**Foundation Run** 5:00 at RPE 2–3 15:00 at RPE 3–4	**Marathon Race**

Marathon

2

Marathon

This plan is designed for serious competitive runners seeking the absolute limit of their potential at the marathon distance. Before starting the plan, be sure to build your training to the point where you're comfortably able to run nine times per week for up to 23 km.

	MONDAY	TUESDAY	WEDNESDAY	THURSDAY
1	**Recovery Run** 40:00 at RPE 2–3	**Progression Run** 5:00 at RPE 2–3 35:00 at RPE 3–4 8:00 at SSP 4:00 at LTP 2:00 at CV 5:00 at RPE 2–3 **Recovery Run** 20:00 at RPE 2–3	**Foundation Run** 5:00 at RPE 2–3 55:00 at RPE 3–4	**Foundation Run** 5:00 at RPE 2–3 55:00 at RPE 3–4
2	**Recovery Run** 40:00 at RPE 2–3	**Progression Run** 5:00 at RPE 2–3 40:00 at RPE 3–4 4:00 at LTP 2:00 at CV 1:00 at MAS 5:00 at RPE 2–3 **Recovery Run** 20:00 at RPE 2–3	**Foundation Run** 5:00 at RPE 2–3 55:00 at RPE 3–4	**Foundation Run** 5:00 at RPE 2–3 55:00 at RPE 3–4
3	Rest	**Progression Run** 5:00 at RPE 2–3 35:00 at RPE 3–4 8:00 at SSP 4:00 at LTP 2:00 at CV 5:00 at RPE 2–3 **Recovery Run** 20:00 at RPE 2–3	**Foundation Run** 5:00 at RPE 2–3 55:00 at RPE 3–4	**Foundation Run** 5:00 at RPE 2–3 55:00 at RPE 3–4

LEVEL

SSP Steady State Pace
LTP Lactate Threshold Pace
CV Critical Velocity
MAS Maximal Aerobic Speed

5KP 5K Pace
HMP Half-Marathon Pace
MP Marathon Pace

FRIDAY

Fartleks
5:00 at RPE 2–3
10:00 at RPE 3–4
8 × 1:00 at RPE 7–8 /
  2:00 at RPE 2–3
15:00 at RPE 3–4

Recovery Run
20:00 at RPE 2–3

Fartleks
5:00 at RPE 2–3
15:00 at RPE 3–4
10 × 0:20 at RPE 8–9 /
  1:40 at RPE 2–3
20:00 at RPE 3–4

Recovery Run
20:00 at RPE 2–3

Fartleks
5:00 at RPE 2–3
10:00 at RPE 3–4
8 × 1:00 at RPE 7–8 /
  2:00 at RPE 2–3
15:00 at RPE 3–4

Recovery Run
20:00 at RPE 2–3

SATURDAY

Foundation Run
5:00 at RPE 2–3
55:00 at RPE 3–4

Foundation Run
5:00 at RPE 2–3
55:00 at RPE 3–4

Foundation Run
5:00 at RPE 2–3
55:00 at RPE 3–4

SUNDAY

Long Run with Fast Finish
1 km at RPE 2–3
21 km at RPE 3–4
1 km at RPE 4–5

Long Run with Fast Finish
1 km at RPE 2–3
25 km at RPE 3–4
1 km at RPE 4–5

Depletion Run
5:00 at RPE 2–3
1:35:00 at RPE 3–4
No calories before or during

Marathon

3

	MONDAY	TUESDAY	WEDNESDAY	THURSDAY

4	**Recovery Run**
	40:00 at RPE 2–3
		Progression Fartleks
		5:00 at RPE 2–3
		15:00 at RPE 3–4
		2 × (3:00 at RPE 4–5 /
		  1:00 at RPE 2–3)
		2 × (4:00 at RPE 5–6 /
		  1:00 at RPE 2–3)
		2 × (5:00 at RPE 6–7 /
		  1:00 at RPE 2–3)
		20:00 at RPE 2–3
		
		Recovery Run
		25:00 at RPE 2–3
			Foundation Run
			5:00 at RPE 2–3
			55:00 at RPE 3–4
				Foundation Run
				5:00 at RPE 2–3
				1:00:00 at RPE 3–4

5	**Recovery Run** 40:00 at RPE 2–3	**Critical Velocity Intervals** 5:00 at RPE 2–3 15:00 at RPE 3–4 7 × 4:00* at RPE 6–7 / 2:00 at RPE 2–3 20:00 at RPE 2–3 *Precision Splitting **Recovery Run** 25:00 at RPE 2–3	**Foundation Run** 5:00 at RPE 2–3 55:00 at RPE 3–4	**Foundation Run** 5:00 at RPE 2–3 1:00:00 at RPE 3–4
6	Rest	**Fartleks** 5:00 at RPE 2–3 15:00 at RPE 3–4 1:00 at CV, 1:00 at RPE 2–3 2:00 at LTP, 1:00 at RPE 2–3 3:00 at SSP, 1:00 at RPE 2–3 2:00 at LTP, 1:00 at RPE 2–3 1:00 at CV, 1:00 at RPE 2–3 2:00 at LTP, 1:00 at RPE 2–3 3:00 at SSP, 1:00 at RPE 2–3 2:00 at LTP, 1:00 at RPE 2–3 1:00 at CV, 1:00 at RPE 2–3 20:00 at RPE 3–4 **Recovery Run** 20:00 at RPE 2–3	**Foundation Run** 5:00 at RPE 2–3 55:00 at RPE 3–4	**Foundation Run** 5:00 at RPE 2–3 55:00 at RPE 3–4
7	**Recovery Run** 40:00 at RPE 2–3	**Steady State Run** 5:00 at RPE 2–3 15:00 at RPE 3–4 50:00 at RPE 5 20:00 at RPE 2–3 **Recovery Run** 30:00 at RPE 2–3	**Foundation Run** 5:00 at RPE 2–3 55:00 at RPE 3–4	**Foundation Run** 5:00 at RPE 2–3 1:05:00 at RPE 3–4
8	**Recovery Run** 40:00 at RPE 2–3	**Tempo Run** 5:00 at RPE 2–3 15:00 at RPE 3–4 18:00 at RPE 6 5:00 at RPE 2–3 18:00 at RPE 6 20:00 at RPE 2–3 **Recovery Run** 30:00 at RPE 2–3	**Foundation Run** 5:00 at RPE 2–3 55:00 at RPE 3–4	**Foundation Run** 5:00 at RPE 2–3 1:05:00 at RPE 3–4

FRIDAY	SATURDAY	SUNDAY
Hill Repetitions	**Foundation Run**	**Half-Marathon Pace Run**
5:00 at RPE 2–3	5:00 at RPE 2–3	1 km at RPE 2–3
15:00 at RPE 3–4	55:00 at RPE 3–4	4 km at RPE 3–4
12 × 0:30 uphill at RPE 8–9 /		3 × (3 km at HMP / 1:00 rest)
1:30 at RPE 2–3		5 km at RPE 2–3
20:00 at RPE 2–3		
Precision Splitting		
Recovery Run		
25:00 at RPE 2–3		
Accelerations	**Foundation Run**	**Long Run with Fast Finish**
5:00 at RPE 2–3	5:00 at RPE 2–3	1 km at RPE 2–3
15:00 at RPE 3–4	55:00 at RPE 3–4	27 km at RPE 3–4
11:00 acceleration		1 km at RPE 4–5
10:00 at RPE 2–3		
6:00 acceleration		
10:00 at RPE 2–3		
11:00 acceleration		
20:00 at RPE 2–3		
Recovery Run		
25:00 at RPE 2–3		
Speed Intervals	**Foundation Run**	**Depletion Run**
5:00 at RPE 2–3	5:00 at RPE 2–3	5:00 at RPE 2–3
15:00 at RPE 3–4	55:00 at RPE 3–4	1:55:00 at RPE 3–4
12 × 0:45* at RPE 8–9 /		*No calories before or during*
1:45 at RPE 2–3		
20:00 at RPE 2–3		
Stretch Intervals		
Recovery Run		
20:00 at RPE 2–3		
VO₂max Intervals	**Foundation Run**	**Long Run with Fast Finish**
5:00 at RPE 2–3	5:00 at RPE 2–3	1 km at RPE 2–3
15:00 at RPE 3–4	55:00 at RPE 3–4	30 km at RPE 3–4
7 × 2:00* at RPE 7–8 /		2 km at RPE 5–6*
1:00 at RPE 2–3		*Note the slightly more aggressive
20:00 at RPE 2–3		fast finish.*
Precision Splitting		
Recovery Run		
30:00 at RPE 2–3		
5K Pace Intervals	**Foundation Run**	**Marathon Pace Run**
1 km at RPE 2–3	5:00 at RPE 2–3	1 km (0.6 mile) at RPE 2–3
4 km at RPE 3–4	55:00 at RPE 3–4	2 km (1.2 miles) at RPE 3–4
6 × (0.8 km at 5KP* / 1:00 rest)		6 × 1.5 km (0.9 mile) at MP /
5 km at RPE 2–3		1.5 km (0.9 mile) at RPE 3–4
Precision Splitting		2 km (1.2 miles) at RPE 2–3
Recovery Run		
30:00 at RPE 2–3		

VO_2

Marathon

3

	MONDAY	TUESDAY	WEDNESDAY	THURSDAY
9	Rest	**Progression Run** 5:00 at RPE 2–3 40:00 at RPE 3–4 4:00 at LTP 2:00 at CV 1:00 at MAS 5:00 at RPE 2–3 **Recovery Run** 25:00 at RPE 2–3	**Foundation Run** 5:00 at RPE 2–3 55:00 at RPE 3–4	**Foundation Run** 5:00 at RPE 2–3 55:00 at RPE 3–4

10	**Recovery Run**
	40:00 at RPE 2–3
		Progression Fartleks
		5:00 at RPE 2–3
		15:00 at RPE 3–4
		2 × (3:00 at RPE 4–5 /
		  1:00 at RPE 2–3)
		2 × (4:00 at RPE 5–6 /
		  1:00 at RPE 2–3)
		2 × (5:00 at RPE 6–7 /
		  1:00 at RPE 2–3)
		2 × (6:00 at RPE 6–7 /
		  1:00 at RPE 2–3)
		20:00 at RPE 2–3
		
		Recovery Run
		35:00 at RPE 2–3
			Foundation Run
			5:00 at RPE 2–3
			55:00 at RPE 3–4
				Foundation Run
				5:00 at RPE 2–3
				1:10:00 at RPE 3–4

11	**Recovery Run** 40:00 at RPE 2–3	**Critical Velocity Intervals** 5:00 at RPE 2–3 15:00 at RPE 3–4 8 × 4:00* at RPE 6–7 / 2:00 at RPE 2–3 20:00 at RPE 2–3 *Precision Splitting* **Recovery Run** 35:00 at RPE 2–3	**Foundation Run** 5:00 at RPE 2–3 55:00 at RPE 3–4	**Foundation Run** 5:00 at RPE 2–3 1:10:00 at RPE 3–4
12	Rest	**Fartleks** 5:00 at RPE 2–3 15:00 at RPE 3–4 1:00 at CV, 1:00 at RPE 2–3 2:00 at LTP, 1:00 at RPE 2–3 3:00 at SSP, 1:00 at RPE 2–3 2:00 at LTP, 1:00 at RPE 2–3 1:00 at CV, 1:00 at RPE 2–3 2:00 at LTP, 1:00 at RPE 2–3 3:00 at SSP, 1:00 at RPE 2–3 2:00 at LTP, 1:00 at RPE 2–3 1:00 at CV, 1:00 at RPE 2–3 20:00 at RPE 3–4 **Recovery Run** 30:00 at RPE 2–3	**Foundation Run** 5:00 at RPE 2–3 55:00 at RPE 3–4	**Foundation Run** 5:00 at RPE 2–3 55:00 at RPE 3–4

FRIDAY	SATURDAY	SUNDAY

Hill Repetitions
5:00 at RPE 2–3
15:00 at RPE 3–4
10 × 1:00 uphill at RPE 8–9* /
   2:00 at RPE 2–3
20:00 at RPE 2–3
Stretch Intervals

Recovery Run
25:00 at RPE 2–3

Foundation Run
5:00 at RPE 2–3
55:00 at RPE 3–4

Long Run with Fast Finish
1 km at RPE 2–3
19 km at RPE 3–4
1 km at RPE 4–5

The Prefontaine
1 km at RPE 2–3
4 km at RPE 3–4
? × 200m at RPE 9 /
   200m at RPE 6
1 km at RPE 2–3
4 km at RPE 3–4
(? = Go to failure)

Recovery Run
35:00 at RPE 2–3

Foundation Run
5:00 at RPE 2–3
55:00 at RPE 3–4

Long Run with Fast Finish
1 km at RPE 2–3
30 km at RPE 3–4
2 km at RPE 5–6*
Note the slightly more aggressive fast finish.

Fartleks
5:00 at RPE 2–3
15:00 at RPE 3–4
10 × 0:20 at RPE 8–9 /
   1:40 at RPE 2–3
20:00 at RPE 3–4

Recovery Run
35:00 at RPE 2–3

Foundation Run
5:00 at RPE 2–3
55:00 at RPE 3–4

Marathon Pace Run
1 km (0.6 mile) at RPE 2–3
2 km (1.2 miles) at RPE 3–4
20 km (12.4 miles) at MP
2 km (1.2 miles) at RPE 2–3

VO$_2$max Intervals
5:00 at RPE 2–3
15:00 at RPE 3–4
6 × 2:00 at RPE 7–8* /
   1:00 at RPE 2–3
20:00 at RPE 2–3
Precision Splitting

Recovery Run
30:00 at RPE 2–3

Foundation Run
5:00 at RPE 2–3
55:00 at RPE 3–4

Depletion Run
5:00 at RPE 2–3
2:15:00 at RPE 3–4
No calories before or during

Marathon

3

	MONDAY	TUESDAY	WEDNESDAY	THURSDAY
13	**Recovery Run** 40:00 at RPE 2–3	**Steady State Run** 5:00 at RPE 2–3 15:00 at RPE 3–4 1:00:00 at RPE 5 20:00 at RPE 2–3 **Recovery Run** 40:00 at RPE 2–3	**Foundation Run** 5:00 at RPE 2–3 55:00 at RPE 3–4	**Foundation Run** 5:00 at RPE 2–3 1:10:00 at RPE 3–4
14	**Recovery Run** 40:00 at RPE 2–3	**Tempo Run** 5:00 at RPE 2–3 15:00 at RPE 3–4 22:00 at RPE 6 5:00 at RPE 2–3 22:00 at RPE 6 20:00 at RPE 2–3 **Recovery Run** 40:00 at RPE 2–3	**Foundation Run** 5:00 at RPE 2–3 55:00 at RPE 3–4	**Foundation Run** 5:00 at RPE 2–3 1:10:00 at RPE 3–4
15	Rest	**Progression Run** 5:00 at RPE 2–3 25:00 at RPE 3–4 16:00 at SSP 8:00 at LTP 4:00 at CV 5:00 at RPE 2–3 **Recovery Run** 30:00 at RPE 2–3	**Foundation Run** 5:00 at RPE 2–3 55:00 at RPE 3–4	**Foundation Run** 5:00 at RPE 2–3 55:00 at RPE 3–4
16	**Recovery Run** 40:00 at RPE 2–3	**Steady State Run** 5:00 at RPE 2–3 15:00 at RPE 3–4 1:10:00 at RPE 5 20:00 at RPE 2–3 **Recovery Run** 40:00 at RPE 2–3	**Foundation Run** 5:00 at RPE 2–3 55:00 at RPE 3–4	**Foundation Run** 5:00 at RPE 2–3 1:10:00 at RPE 3–4
17	**Recovery Run** 40:00 at RPE 2–3	**Relaxed 10K Time Trial** 1 km at RPE 2–3 4 km at RPE 3–4 10 km at 95% effort 5 km at RPE 2–3 **Recovery Run** 30:00 at RPE 2–3	**Foundation Run** 5:00 at RPE 2–3 55:00 at RPE 3–4	**Foundation Run** 5:00 at RPE 2–3 55:00 at RPE 3–4
18	Rest	**Fartleks** 5:00 at RPE 2–3 15:00 at RPE 3–4 10 × 1:00 at RPE 7–8 / 2:00 at RPE 2–3 20:00 at RPE 3–4	**Foundation Run** 5:00 at RPE 2–3 40:00 at RPE 3–4	**Foundation Run** 5:00 at RPE 2–3 40:00 at RPE 3–4

FRIDAY	SATURDAY	SUNDAY
5K Pace Intervals 1 km at RPE 2–3 4 km at RPE 3–4 8 × (0.6 km at 5KP* / 1:00 rest) 5 km at RPE 2–3 *Precision Splitting* **Recovery Run** 40:00 at RPE 2–3	**Foundation Run** 5:00 at RPE 2–3 55:00 at RPE 3–4	**Marathon Pace Run** 1 km at RPE 2–3 15 km at RPE 3–4 16 km at MP
Relaxed 5K Time Trial 1 km at RPE 2–3 4 km at RPE 3–4 5 km at 95% effort 5 km at RPE 2–3 **Recovery Run** 40:00 at RPE 2–3	**Foundation Run** 5:00 at RPE 2–3 55:00 at RPE 3–4	**Long Run with Fast Finish** 1 km at RPE 2–3 32 km at RPE 3–4 2 km at RPE 5–6* *Note the slightly more aggressive fast finish.*
Hill Repetitions 5:00 at RPE 2–3 15:00 at RPE 3–4 6 × 2:00 at RPE 7–8* / 2:00 at RPE 2–3 20:00 at RPE 2–3 *Stretch Intervals* **Recovery Run** 30:00 at RPE 2–3	**Foundation Run** 5:00 at RPE 2–3 55:00 at RPE 3–4	**Depletion Run** 5:00 at RPE 2–3 2:35:00 at RPE 3–4 *No calories before or during*
Speed Intervals 5:00 at RPE 2–3 15:00 at RPE 3–4 10 × 1:00* at RPE 8–9 / 2:00 at RPE 2–3 20:00 at RPE 2–3 *Stretch Intervals* **Recovery Run** 40:00 at RPE 2–3	**Foundation Run** 5:00 at RPE 2–3 55:00 at RPE 3–4	**Marathon Pace Run** 1 km (0.6 mile) at RPE 2–3 2 km (1.2 miles) at RPE 3–4 26 km (16.1 miles) at MP 2 km (1.2 miles) at RPE 2–3
VO$_2$max Intervals 5:00 at RPE 2–3 15:00 at RPE 3–4 6 × 2:00 at RPE 7–8* / 1:00 at RPE 2–3 20:00 at RPE 2–3 *Precision Splitting* **Recovery Run** 30:00 at RPE 2–3	**Foundation Run** 5:00 at RPE 2–3 55:00 at RPE 3–4	**Long Run with Fast Finish** 1 km at RPE 2–3 16 km at RPE 3–4 2 km at RPE 5–6* *Note the slightly more aggressive fast finish.*
Fast Finish Run 5:00 at RPE 2–3 20:00 at RPE 3–4 10:00 at RPE 6	**Foundation Run** 5:00 at RPE 2–3 15:00 at RPE 3–4	**Marathon Race**

Marathon

3

References

Chapter 2

Farrell, P. A., J. H. Wilmore, E. F. Coyle, J.E. Billing, and D. L. Costill. "Plasma Lactate Accumulation and Distance Running Performance." *Medicine & Science in Sports & Exercise* 11, 4 (1979): 338–44.

Marcora, Samuele M. "Do We Really Need a Central Governor to Explain Brain Regulation of Exercise Performance?" *European Journal of Applied Physiology* 104, 5 (November 2008): 929–31.

Marcora, Samuele M., and Walter Staiano. "The Limit to Exercise Tolerance in Humans: Mind Over Muscle?" *European Journal of Applied Physiology* 109, 4 (July 2010): 763–70.

Mauger Alexis R., and Nick Sculthorpe. "A New VO_2max Protocol Allowing Self-Pacing in Maximal Incremental Exercise." *British Journal of Sports Medicine* 46, 1 (January 2012): 59–63.

Morales-Alamo, David, José Losa-Reyna, Rafael Torres-Peralta, Marcos Martin-Rincon, Mario Perez-Valera, David Curtelin, Jesús Gustavo Ponce-González, Alfredo Santana, and José A. L. Calbet. "What Limits Performance During Whole-Body Incremental Exercise to Exhaustion in Humans?" *Journal of Physiology* 593, 20 (October 2015): 4631–48.

Viana, Bruno Ferreira, Flávio Oliveira Pires, Allan Inoue, Dominic Micklewright, and Tony Meireles Santos. "Correlates of Mood and RPE During Multi-Lap Off-Road Cycling." *Applied Psychophysiology and Biofeedback* 41, 1 (March 2016): 1–7.

Chapter 3

Bayne, Freya, Sebastien Racinais, Katya Mileva, Steve Hunter, and Nadia Gaoua. "Less Is More-Cyclists-Triathlete's 30 min Cycling Time-Trial Performance Is Impaired with Multiple Feedback Compared to a Single Feedback." *Frontiers in Psychology* 11 (December 2020): 608426.

Boya, Manhal, Tom Foulsham, Florentina Hettinga, David Parry, Emily Williams, Hollie Jones, Andrew Sparks, David Marchant, Paul Ellison, Craig Bridge, Lars McNaughton, and Dominic Micklewright. "Information Acquisition Differences Between Experienced and Novice Time Trial Cyclists." *Medicine & Science in Sports & Exercise* 49, 9 (September 2017): 1884–98.

Crawley, Michael. *Out of Thin Air: Running Wisdom and Magic from Above the Clouds in Ethiopia*. London: Bloomsbury, 2020.

Diotaiuti, Pierluigi, Stefania Mancone, and Stefano Corrado. "Using Sports Tracker: Evidences on Dependence, Self-Regulatory Modes and Resilience in a Sample of Competitive Runners." *Psychology* 11, 1 (January 2020): 54–70.

Garcin, Murielle, Jérémy B. J. Coquart, Sophie Robin, and Régis Matran. "Prediction of Time to Exhaustion in Competitive Cyclists from a Perceptually Based Scale. *s* 25, 5 (May 2011): 1393–9.

Karahanoğlu, Armagan, Rúben Gouveia, Jasper Reenalda, and Geke Ludden. "How Are Sports-Trackers Used by Runners? Running-Related Data, Personal Goals, and Self-Tracking in Running." *Sensors* 21, 11 (2021): 3687.

Lambrick, Danielle, Alex Rowlands, Thomas Rowland, and Roger G. Eston. "Pacing Strategies of Inexperienced Children During Repeated 800 m Individual Time-Trials and Simulated Competition." *Pediatric Exercise Science* 25, 2 (May 2013): 198–211.

Latorre-Román, Pedro Ángel, Juan Francisco Fernández-Povedano, Jesús Salas-Sánchez, Felipe García-Pinillos, and Juan Antonio Párraga-Montilla. "The Ability of Runners to Identify Spatial and Temporal Variables of Speed During Endurance Running." *Motor Control* 24, 4 (July 2020): 499–511.

Nikolaidis, Pantelis T., and Beat Knechtle. "Pacing in Age Group Marathoners in the 'New York City Marathon.'" *Research in Sports Medicine* 26, 1 (January–March 2018): 86–99.

Walsh, Vincent. "Is Sport the Brain's Biggest Challenge?" *Current Biology* 24, 18 (September 2014): R859–R860.

Chapter 4

Cona, Giorgia, Annachiara Cavazzana, Antonio Paoli, Giuseppe Marcolin, Alessandro Grainer, and Patrizia Silvia Bisiacchi. "It's a Matter of Mind! Cognitive Functioning Predicts the Athletic Performance in Ultra-Marathon Runners." *PLOS One* 10, 7 (July 2015): e0132943.

Edwards, Andrew, and Remco Polman. *Pacing in Sport and Exercise: A Psychophysiological Perspective*. New York: Nova, 2012.

Elbert, T., C. Pantev, C. Wienbruch, B. Rockstroh, and E. Taub. "Increased Cortical Representation of the Fingers of the Left Hand in String Players." *Science* 270, 5234 (October 1995): 305–7.

Elferink-Gemser, Marije T., and Florentina J. Hettinga. "Pacing and Self-Regulation: Important Skills for Talent Development in Endurance Sports." *International Journal of Sports Physiology and Performance* 12, 6 (July 2017): 831–35.

Eskreis-Winkler, Lauren, James J. Gross, and Angela L. Duckworth. "Grit: Sustained Self-Regulation in the Service of Superordinate Goals." In *Handbook of Self-Regulation: Research, Theory and Applications,* 3rd ed., edited by Kathleen D. Vohs and Roy F. Baumeister. New York: Guilford, 2016.

Herbert, Beate M., Pamela Ulbrich, and Rainer Schandry. "Interoceptive Sensitivity and Physical Effort: Implications for the Self-Control of Physical Load in Everyday Life." *Psychophysiology* 44, 2 (March 2007): 194–202.

Hirsh, Jacob B. "Decision-Making and Self-Regulation from a Social-Personality Neuroscience Perspective." Unpublished doctoral thesis. University of Toronto, 2010. https://tspace. library.utoronto.ca/bitstream/1807/32936/3/Hirsh_Jacob_B_20106_PhD_thesis.pdf.

Lee, Tatia M. C., Chetwyn C. H. Chan, Ada W. S. Leung, Peter T. Fox, and Jia-Hong Gao. "Sex-Related Differences in Neural Activity During Risk Taking: An fMRI Study." *Cerebral Cortex* 19, 6 (June 2009): 1303–12.

Liew, Guo Chen, Garry Kuan, Ngien Siong Chin, and Hairul Anuar Hashim. "Mental Toughness in Sport." *German Journal of Exercise and Sport Research* 49 (2019): 381–94.

Méndez-Alonso, David, Jose Antonio Prieto-Saborit, Jose Ramón Bahamonde, and Estíbaliz Jiménez-Arberás. "Influence of Psychological Factors on the Success of the Ultra-Trail Runner. *International Journal of Environmental Research and Public Health* 18, 5 (March 2021): 2704.

Scruton, Adrian, James Baker, Justin Roberts, Itay Basevitch, Viviane Merzbach, and Dan Gordon. "Pacing Accuracy During an Incremental Step Test in Adolescent Swimmers." *Open Access Journal of Sports Medicine* 6 (2015): 249–57.

Skorski, S., O. Faude, K. Rausch, and T. Meyer. "Reproducibility of Pacing Profiles in Competitive Swimmers." *International Journal of Sports Medicine* 34, 2 (February 2013): 152–57.

Smyth, Barry, and Aonghus Lawlor. "Longer Disciplined Tapers Improve Marathon Performance for Recreational Runners." *Frontiers in Sports and Active Living* 3 (September 2021): 735220.

Wiersma, Rikstje, Inge K. Stoter, Chris Visscher, Florentina J. Hettinga, and Marije T. Elferink-Gemser. "Development of 1500-m Pacing Behavior in Junior Speed Skaters: A Longitudinal Study." *International Journal of Sports Physiology and Performance* 12, 9 (October 2017): 1224–31.

Chapter 5

Blanchfield, Anthony William, James Hardy, Helma Majella De Morree, Walter Staiano, and Samuele Maria Marcora. "Talking Yourself Out of Exhaustion: The Effects of Self-Talk on Endurance Performance." *Medicine & Science in Sports & Exercise* 46, 5 (2014): 998–1007.

Brick, Noel, Mark J. Campbell, and Tadhg Macintyre. "Metacognitive Processes in the Self-Regulation of Performance in Elite Distance Runners." *Psychology of Sport and Exercise* 19 (February 2015): 1–9.

Crust, Lee, and Peter J. Clough. "Developing Mental Toughness: From Research to Practice." *Journal of Sport Psychology in Action* 2, 1 (2011): 21–32.

do Carmo, Everton C., Renato Barroso, Andrew Renfree, Natalia R. da Silva, Saulo Gil, and Valmor Tricoli. "Affective Feelings and Perceived Exertion During a 10-km Time Trial and Head-to-Head Running Race." *International Journal of Sports Physiology and Performance* 11 (February 2020): 1–4.

García-González, Luis, M. Perla Moreno, Alberto Moreno, Alexander Gil, and Fernando del Villar. "Effectiveness of a Video-Feedback and Questioning Programme to Develop Cognitive Expertise in Sport." *PLOS One* 8, 12 (2013): e82270.

Murakami, Haruki. *What I Talk About When I Talk About Running: A Memoir.* New York: Vintage, 2008.

O'Leary, Thomas J., Johnny Collett, Ken Howells, and Martyn G. Morris. "High But Not Moderate-Intensity Endurance Training Increases Pain Tolerance: A Randomised Trial." *European Journal of Applied Physiology* 117, 11 (November 2017): 2201–10.

Chapter 6

Borg, G. A. "Psychophysical Bases of Perceived Exertion." *Medicine & Science in Sports & Exercise* 14, 5 (1982): 377–81.

Scherr, Johannes, Bernd Wolfarth, Jeffrey W. Christle, Axel Pressler, Stefan Wagenpfeil, and Martin Halle. "Associations Between Borg's Rating of Perceived Exertion and Physiological Measures of Exercise Intensity." *European Journal of Applied Physiology* 113, 1 (January 2013): 147–55.

"Sport and Study a Winning Combination." Sportaus, August 5, 2016. https://www.sportaus. gov.au/media-centre/news/sport_and_study_a_winning_combination.

Chapter 7

Wiggins, Bradley. *My Hour.* London: Vintage, 2015.

About the Author

Matt Fitzgerald is a prolific endurance sports author, coach, and nutritionist. His many books include *The Comeback Quotient*, *80/20 Running*, and *The Endurance Diet*. Matt has also written training and feature articles for the leading sports media brands, including *Runner's World* and *Triathlete*, and for popular websites such as outsideonline.com and nbcnews.com. He is cofounder of 80/20 Endurance, where athletes can access training plans, videos, and other invaluable resources and

inspiration, including a regular 80/20 Endurance podcast and blog. He also codirects the Coaches of Color Initiative, a nonprofit program that seeks to improve diversity in endurance coaching. A lifelong endurance athlete, Matt speaks frequently at events throughout the United States and internationally.

CPSIA information can be obtained
at www.ICGtesting.com
Printed in the USA
BVHW031354170922
647223BV00015B/1108